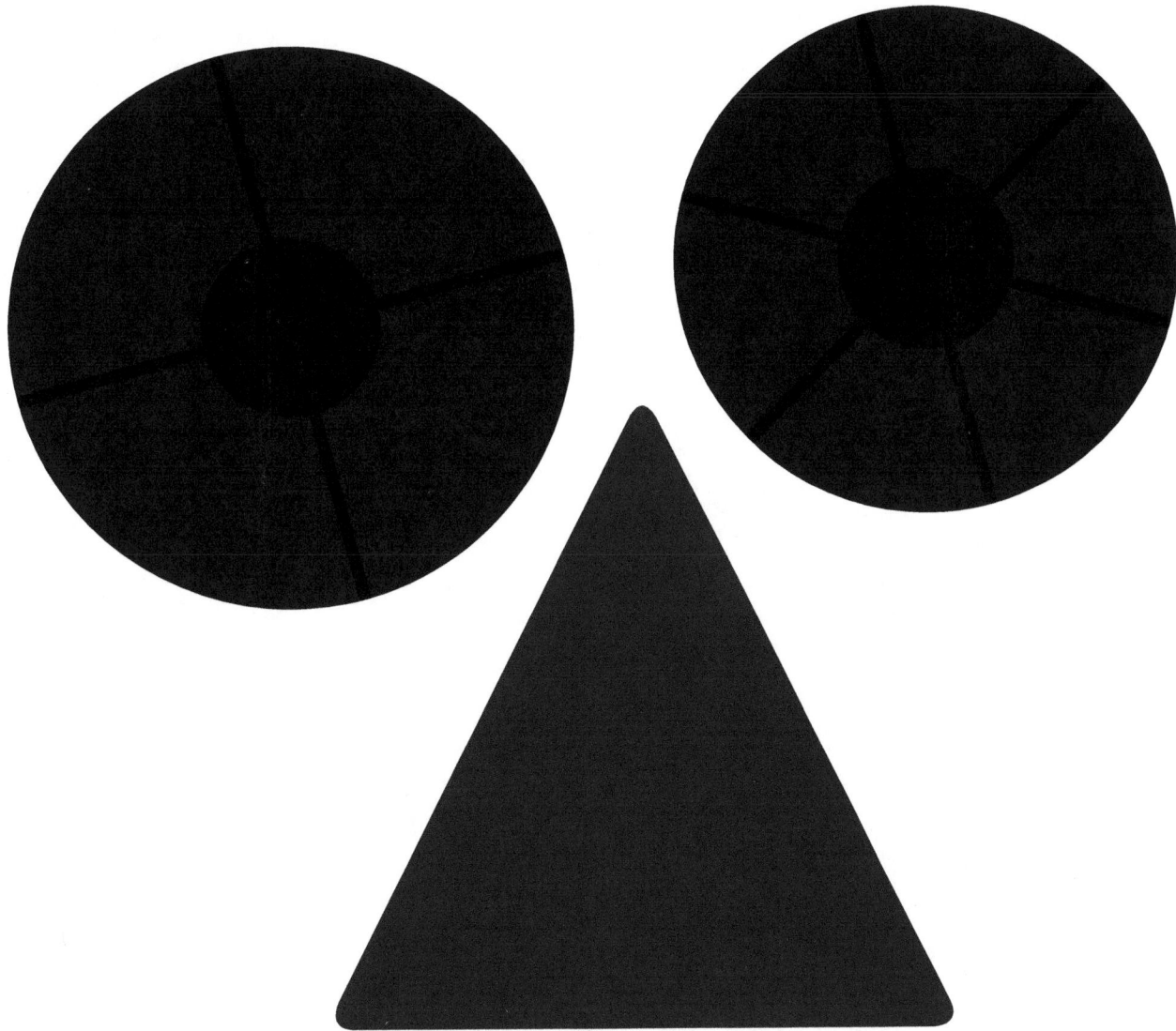

The Face of Wellness

A Conceptual Framework to Guide the Development of Effective Health Promotion Programs: The Awareness, Motivation, Skills and Opportunity (AMSO) Framework and the Face of Wellness Model

Michael P. O'Donnell MBA, MPH, PhD

This workbook is published by the American Journal of Health Promotion. P.O. Box 1254, Troy, Michigan 48099-1254. Some of the contents are excerpted from Health Promotion in the Workplace, 4th Edition, to be published in 2014. For additional information about the 4th Edition e-mail contact@healthpromotionjournal.com.

The Face of Wellness

A Conceptual Framework to Guide the
Development of Effective Health Promotion
Programs: The Awareness, Motivation, Skills
and Opportunity (AMSO) Framework
and the Face of Wellness Model

Michael P. O'Donnell MBA, MPH, PhD

AMERICAN JOURNAL *of*

Health Promotion

Table of Contents

I. Process used to Develop the AMSO Framework and Face of Wellness Model..........1

II. The Face of Wellness Model 1

III. An Aspirational Vision of Health...3

IV. Dimensions of Optimal Health..4

V. Renewing Health Behavior Change Process 10

    a. Step 1. Get Ready..12

    b. Step 2. Measure Your Health..13

    c. Step 3. Set Goals..13

    d. Step 4. Build Skills 16

    e. Step 5. Form Habits 18

    f. Step 6. Help Others 19

VI. Awareness, Motivation, Skills and Opportunities 21

    a. Awareness...21

    b. Motivation..22

    c. Skills 26

    d. Opportunity 26

VII. POSSE[2]: The Dimensions of Opportunity...30

    a. P: Peers...30

    b. O: Organizations 31

    c. S: State..32

    d. S: Society 34

    e. E: Environment..35

    f. E: Equality..36

VIII. Relative Importance of Different Strategies...37

IX. Conclusion and Implications..37

X. Appendix A: Historical Roots of an Aspirational Vision of Health 39

XI. Appendix B: Causes of Income Inequality in the United States
and Resulting Health Effects..43

XII. References...49

XIII. About the Author...57

Thi workbook is organized around the Awareness, Motivation, Skills and Opportunity (AMSO) Framework (Framework), which is a component of the Face of Wellness Model (Model). It starts with a review of the process used to develop the Framework and the Model. Next, the three major components of the Model are briefly reviewed: Aspirational Vision of Health, Health Behavior Change Process, and the AMSO Framework. The description of the AMSO Framework includes discussions of the four basic components of the Framework: awareness, motivation, skills and opportunity, and the six components of opportunity: peers, organizations, the state, society, environment and equality.

Process used to Develop the AMSO Framework and Face of Wellness Model

The AMSO Framework and Face of Wellness Model were developed based on a twenty-year quest to answer the question "What works best in workplace health promotion?" The systematic portion of the quest included a benchmarking study that involved collecting basic information on 76 **workplace health promotion programs** that had reported the health and financial impact of their programs in the peer-reviewed literature; additional detail collected through questionnaires on 26 of those programs and more complete information gathered through site visits to the six deemed best practice;[1] a systematic review of the literature on the health impact of workplace health promotion that synthesized the findings of 384 studies[2] and resulted in publication of more than 20 articles;[3,4] plus a systematic review of the literature on the financial impact of workplace health promotion programs that synthesized findings of 72 studies.[5] The non-systematic portion of the process included completing in-depth reviews of more than 2000 articles submitted to the *American Journal of Health Promotion* between 1986 and 2012, reviewing descriptions of more than 200 workplace health promotion programs submitted with applications for the C. Everett Koop Award[6] between 1994 and 2012, and being involved in the design and/or management of programs at more than 50 employers.

The Face of Wellness Model

The image of a face (Figure 1) was chosen to provide a simple and memorable image to organize the principles gleaned from this quest. This image also reminds health promotion

The face of Wellness
A Conceptual Framework to Guide the Development of Effective Health Promotion Programs:
The Awareness, Motivation, Skills and Opportunity (AMSO) Framework and The Face of Wellness Model

professionals that the core of what they do is not about theoretical concepts, analytic methods, budgets, incentives or equipment. It is about people. It is about understanding people's priorities and helping them change in ways that profoundly impact their lives. As the health promotion field becomes more complex, as it depends more on computer technology to deliver programs, as programs are pressured to show a positive *return on investment*, it is easy to forget that the core of health promotion is helping people in very personal ways.

Figure 1

The Face of Wellness: An Integrated Model for Planning Wellness Programs

©2006, Michael P. O'Donnell MBA, MPH, PhD

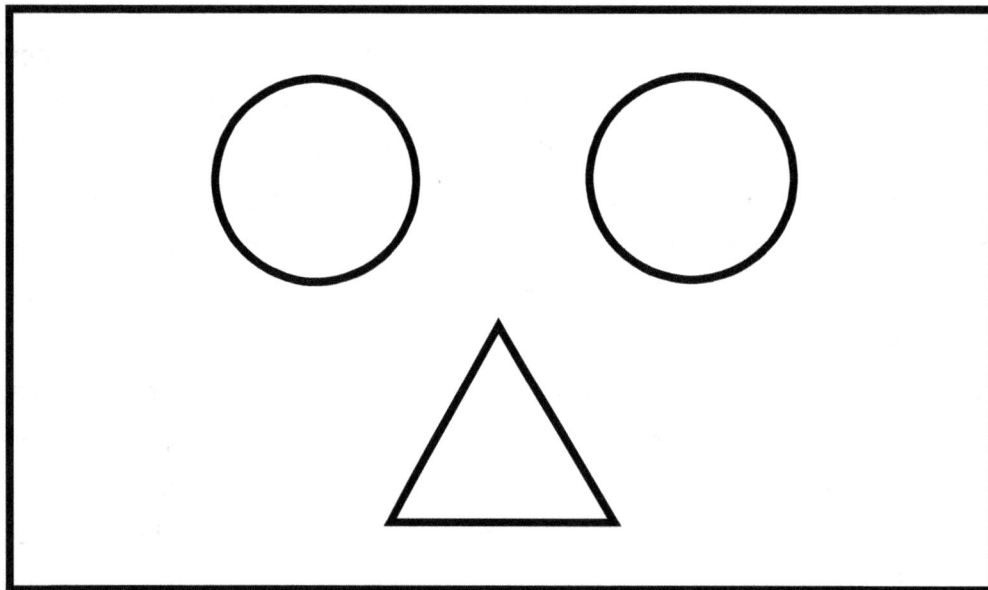

The Face of Wellness model has three basic components: [1] an *Aspirational Vision of Health*, [2] a *Renewing Health Behavior Change Process*, and [3] a *Portfolio Balancing Approach to Planning Change Strategies*. The two eyes represent the Aspirational Vision of Health and the Renewing Health Behavior Change Process, while the nose represents the Portfolio Balancing Approach to Planning Change Strategies. These components are described in detail below.

An Aspirational Vision of Health

Many health promotion professionals (including the author) are health nuts. We want to be physically fit. We eat a nutritious diet. We work at being effective in managing stress. We manage weight consistently. We would never consider using tobacco or putting any abusive substances in our bodies. We want to be healthy because we want to be healthy. We are a bit unusual in this regard, but often do not realize we are unusual. For us, health is the reward in and of itself. Not everyone feels that way.

Health nuts are like money nuts. Money nuts like to make money because they like to make money. Most other people work to make money so they can provide for their family, do fun things, help other people, or feel proud of themselves. Health nuts want to be healthy because they want to be healthy, while most other people who make a point of taking care of their health do so because it leads to other rewards. The more typical person might maintain good health to be a good role model for their kids, to allow them to work hard in a job, to make sure they are alive to see kids and grandkids reach important milestones, to be good at a sport, to look good, to excel at whatever is important to them in life. For example, I have a friend who works out two hours a day, six months a year and eats a nutritious diet because he spends the other six months living in remote parts of the world, hiking through pristine wilderness areas to study fish that have not been exposed to human influences. He is a fish nut. He maintains great health so he can study fish.

The mistake many health promotion professionals make is that they do not realize they themselves are health nuts. When they talk to people about health, they assume others care about health. Sometimes, maybe even most of the time, the people they speak to about health do not care about health – not as much as the health nut cares. When a teenage daughter talks to her dad about music groups, he tries to be polite, but he really doesn't care about the latest teen sensation. When a sports nut talks to a co-worker about basketball stars, the co-worker tries to be polite, but usually doesn't really care about the latest MVP. When a lawn nut talks to a neighbor about his lawn, the neighbor tries to be polite, but really doesn't care about the latest fertilizer mix. Get the idea? When people listen to health promotion professionals talk about health, much of the time they are just being polite; often they really don't care.

The face of Wellness
A Conceptual Framework to Guide the Development of Effective Health Promotion Programs:
The Awareness, Motivation, Skills and Opportunity (AMSO) Framework and The Face of Wellness Model

For this reason, health promotion professionals have more success in reaching people when they think and talk about health in very broad terms. This led me to defining optimal health as "a balance of physical, emotional, social, spiritual, and intellectual health"[7] when the *American Journal of Health Promotion* was launched in 1986. These five dimensions of optimal health are briefly described in Table 1. Most organizations have focused their programs on the physical and emotional dimension, but some have addressed all five areas. Note: See appendix A for brief comments on the historical roots of this aspirational vision.

Table 1

Dimensions of Optimal Health

Physical Health is the condition of your body. Programs include fitness, nutrition, weight control, quitting smoking, alcohol and drug abuse prevention and medical self-care.

Emotional Health is the ability to cope with or avoid stress and other emotional challenges. Programs include employee assistance programs (EAP), stress management, and programs to enhance happiness.

Social Health is the ability to form and maintain nurturing and productive relationships with family, friends, co-workers, neighbors and others. Programs can include training in parenting, conflict resolution, assertiveness and other skill building areas, as well as opportunities for employees to get to know each other in fun social activities and to serve others through volunteer projects.

Intellectual Health encompasses achievements in academics, career, hobbies and cultural pursuits. Programs can include job-focused mentoring and skill enhancement programs, as well as more broadly focused tuition reimbursement policies, book clubs, and cultural outings.

> **Spiritual Health** is having a sense of purpose, love, hope, peace and charity. For some people, this is drawn from being part of an organized religious group; for others, it is having a sense of values inspired by other influences. Programs can include workshops to help people clarify life priorities and set goals as well as allowing people to embrace their religious beliefs.

This broad definition of optimal health is scientifically reasonable because there are compelling links between each of these dimensions and medically based measures of morbidity and mortality. Equally important, this broad definition is engaging to many lay people because it encompasses the elements of life that are typically important to them. This broad definition is inspirational or aspirational because it provides a vision of what might be. It stimulates thinking about personal growth. This is in contrast to compliance-oriented definitions that focus on limiting consumption of certain foods, maintaining a certain weight, exercising a certain number of minutes per week – in other words, directions for reducing "risk" factors.

Over time, it has become clear to professionals who use this definition that it is very difficult to know when one has achieved "balance" among the dimensions. It is also clear that different dimensions are more important to people at different times in their lives. People sometimes need to focus virtually all of their attention on their work (intellectual dimension) to complete an important project. Other times they need to focus time on family members (social) to help others through crucial periods. Other times they need to learn new strategies to help themselves through stressful circumstances (emotional). Even the most dedicated fitness nut and most conscious eater (physical), needs to be reminded to go to the doctor for preventive checkups. Most people need to step back periodically to reflect on what, indeed, is important in life, and get back on track (spiritual). Optimal health is not a static condition; it is a dynamic condition. It is not realistic to expect to reach that magic point of perfect balance and stay there. It is more realistic to seek opportunities for growth and think in terms of a process of *striving* for balance under changing circumstances. Recognizing this, the *American Journal of Health Promotion* revised its definition of optimal health definition to reflect these circumstances. Table 2 shows the original and revised definitions of health promotion and optimal health.

The face of Wellness
A Conceptual Framework to Guide the Development of Effective Health Promotion Programs:
The Awareness, Motivation, Skills and Opportunity (AMSO) Framework and The Face of Wellness Model

Table 2

Evolving Definitions of Health Promotion and Optimal Health

Original Definition

"Health promotion is the science and art of helping people change their lifestyle to move toward a state of optimal health. Optimal health is defined as a balance of physical, emotional, social, spiritual, and intellectual health. Lifestyle change can be facilitated through a combination of efforts to enhance awareness, change behavior and create environments that support good health practices." (O'Donnell, *American Journal of Health Promotion*, 1986, 1, 1, 1)

1989 Revision

"Health promotion is the science and art of helping people change their lifestyle to move toward a state of optimal health. Optimal health is defined as a balance of physical, emotional, social, spiritual, and intellectual health. Lifestyle change can be facilitated through a combination of efforts to enhance awareness, change behavior and create environments that support good health practices. Of the three, supportive environments will probably have the greatest impact in producing lasting change." (O'Donnell, *American Journal of Health Promotion*, 1989, 3, 3, 5)

2008 Revision

"Health promotion is the science and art of helping people change their lifestyle to move toward a state of optimal health. Optimal health is the process of striving for a dynamic balance of physical, emotional, social, spiritual, and intellectual health and discovering the synergies between core passions and each of those dimensions. Lifestyle change can be facilitated through a combination of efforts to enhance awareness, increase motivation, build skills and most importantly, to provide opportunities for positive health practices." (O'Donnell, *American Journal of Health Promotion*, 2008, 23, 2, iv-v)

Table 2 continued

2009 Revision
....

"Health Promotion is the art and science of helping people discover the synergies between their core passions and optimal health, enhancing their motivation to strive for optimal health, and supporting them in changing their lifestyle to move toward a state of optimal health. Optimal health is a dynamic balance of physical, emotional, social, spiritual, and intellectual health. Lifestyle change can be facilitated through a combination of learning experiences that enhance awareness, increase motivation, and build skills and, most important, through the creation of opportunities that open access to environments that make positive health practices the easiest choice." (O'Donnell MP American Journal of Health Promotion, 2009, 24, 1, iv-iv)

People are more likely to strive for growth in each of the dimensions when they discover synergies between those dimensions and their personal passions. If a person's passion is to be a super athlete (physical), s/he can achieve that passion faster by embracing other dimensions of the model. S/he can engage a great coach to provide guidance and teammates for competition (social). S/he can learn how to harness failures and successes to push through challenges (emotional). S/he can learn more about physiology and the mechanics of motion (intellectual) to perfect technique. S/he can also work to understand how athletic aspirations can fit within broader life goals (spiritual). If a person's passion is to be a great parent (social), s/he needs to model nutritious eating habits and physical activity (physical) for children. S/he also needs to know how to keep his or her cool when children are misbehaving (emotional). S/he needs to know when and how to draw on other people for support (social), learn about effective parent skills (intellectual), and help children discover their own priorities in life (spiritual).

People are much more likely to be open to health messages when health promotion professionals help them discover their true passions and help them understand how the other dimensions of health can help them realize these passions. For this reason, one of the five dimensions of optimal health is placed at the center of the illustration (Figure 2). Placing physical health at the center is the default, because physical health is most closely aligned with

The face of Wellness
A Conceptual Framework to Guide the Development of Effective Health Promotion Programs:
The Awareness, Motivation, Skills and Opportunity (AMSO) Framework and The Face of Wellness Model

medically inspired measures of health. This illustration will be most compatible with medically driven health promotion programs. However, the concept might be more engaging to each of the many individuals in an organization if each person is encouraged to put the dimension that best encompasses their passions in the center (Figure 3). Some organizations will choose to feature these five dimensions as central tenants of their programs and will offer specific opportunities to support each dimension. Other organizations will feel that this framework is not sufficiently scientific to feature it broadly, but will use it as an under girder to help them understand their population's needs.

Figure 2

Aspirational Vision of Health with Focus on Physical Health

©2007, Michael P. O'Donnell MBA, MPH, PhD

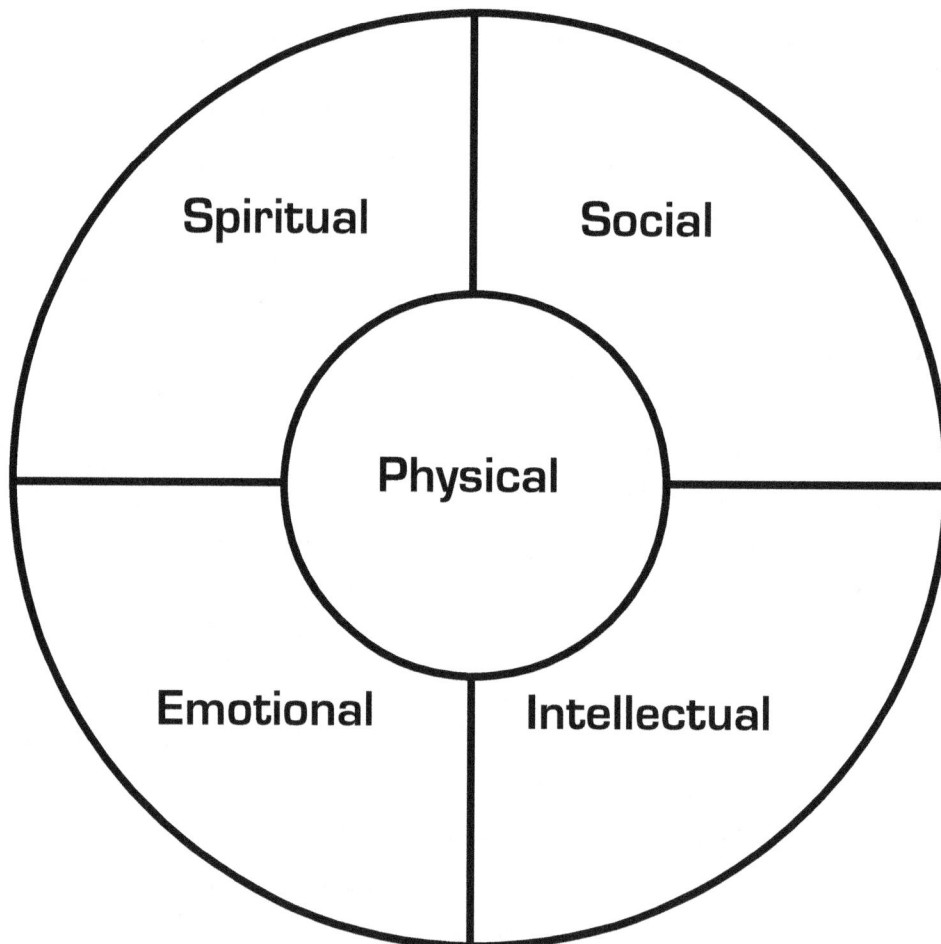

These five dimensions allow a nice balance of parsimony and comprehensiveness and they align well with the types of programs that can be provided in a health promotion program. However, other aspirational definitions of health may work just as well or better for other groups. See definitions from the YMCA, World health Organization and National Wellness Institute in Table 3. Additional dimensions that might be added include environmental sustainability and sexuality.

Figure 3

Aspirational Vision of Health with Focus on Each of the Core Dimensions

©2007, Michael P. O'Donnell MBA, MPH, PhD

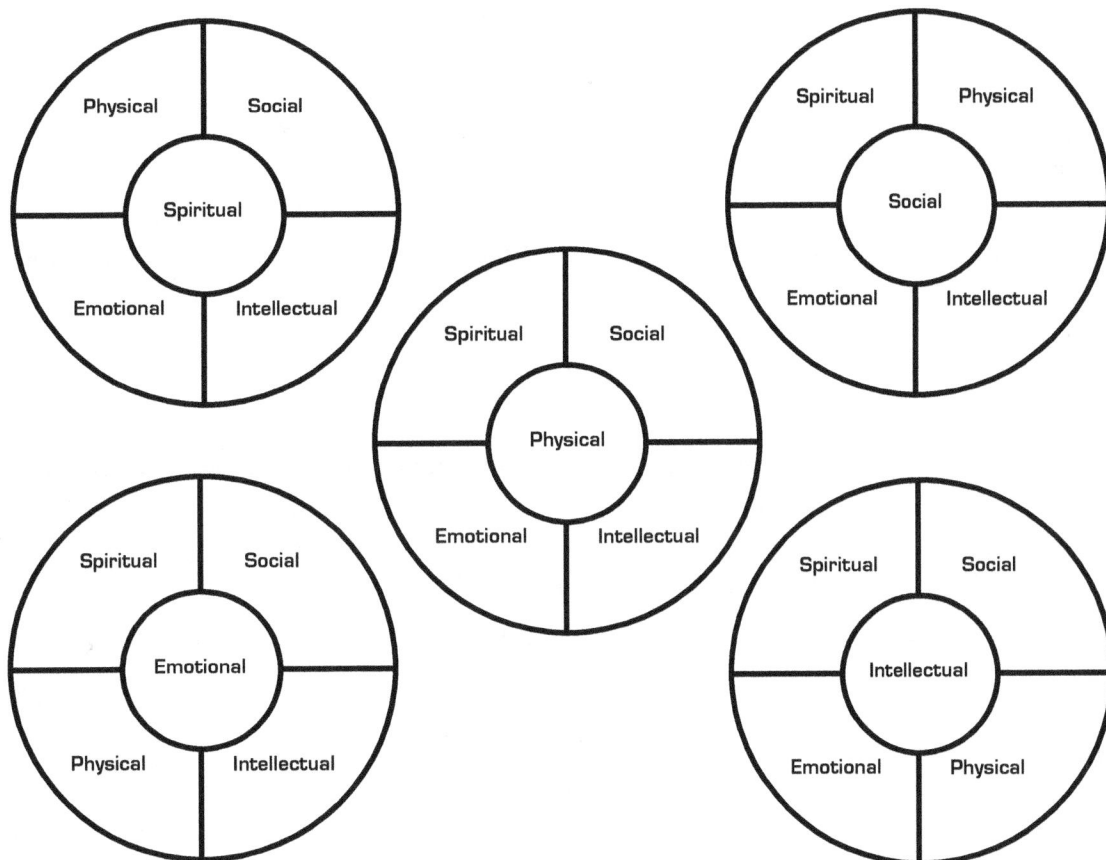

The face of Wellness
A Conceptual Framework to Guide the Development of Effective Health Promotion Programs:
The Awareness, Motivation, Skills and Opportunity (AMSO) Framework and The Face of Wellness Model

Table 3

Other Aspirational Definitions of Health

World Health Organization
· ·

"Health is a state of complete physical, mental and social well-being and not merely the absence of disease or infirmity."

Source: Constitution of the World Health Organization, available at: http://www.who.int

National Wellness Institute
· ·

"Six Dimensions Model: Physical, social, intellectual, spiritual, emotional, occupational"

Source: National Wellness Website. Available at: http://www.nationalwellness.org

YMCA
· ·

"To put Christian principles in to practice through programs that build healthy spirit, mind and body for all."

Source: YMCA website. Available at: http://www.ymca.net

Regardless of the definition of health, the key is helping people discover their life passions and the synergies between those passions and each of the dimensions of optimal health.

Renewing Health Behavior Change Process

Health promotion programs typically engage people in lifestyle change by offering lifestyle questionnaires (*health risk assessments*) and *biomedical screenings* that identify health risk factors and help employees understand the link between lifestyle and health. The next step is to recruit employees into educational and activity programs to support these changes. The more systematic the program offerings, the more likely employees are to follow

10

through. The six-step Renewing Health Behavior Change Process provides a structured approach to doing this. The usual approach is to encourage people to start at the first step and progress through each step sequentially, because this provides a logical approach to change. However, each person needs to be able to start where they are ready to start. Some people start in the middle or the end with no intention of following a set sequence, but eventually realize the wisdom of the sequential process. The goal in offering programs should be to help people eventually cover as many of the steps as possible. The six steps are listed and described below and illustrated (Figure 4). The process renews annually or when people are ready to adopt a new health habit. The steps in this process were inspired by a different but similar set of strategies developed by StayWell Health Management in the early1980s.[8] These steps are similar to 12 step models used in addiction recovery programs.[9]

1. Get ready

2. Measure your health

3. Set goals

4. Build skills

5. Form habits

6. Help others

One of the keys to success in this process is to include activities in each step that stimulate the person to move to the next step.

The face of Wellness
A Conceptual Framework to Guide the Development of Effective Health Promotion Programs:
The Awareness, Motivation, Skills and Opportunity (AMSO) Framework and The Face of Wellness Model

Figure 4

Renewing Health Behavior Change Process

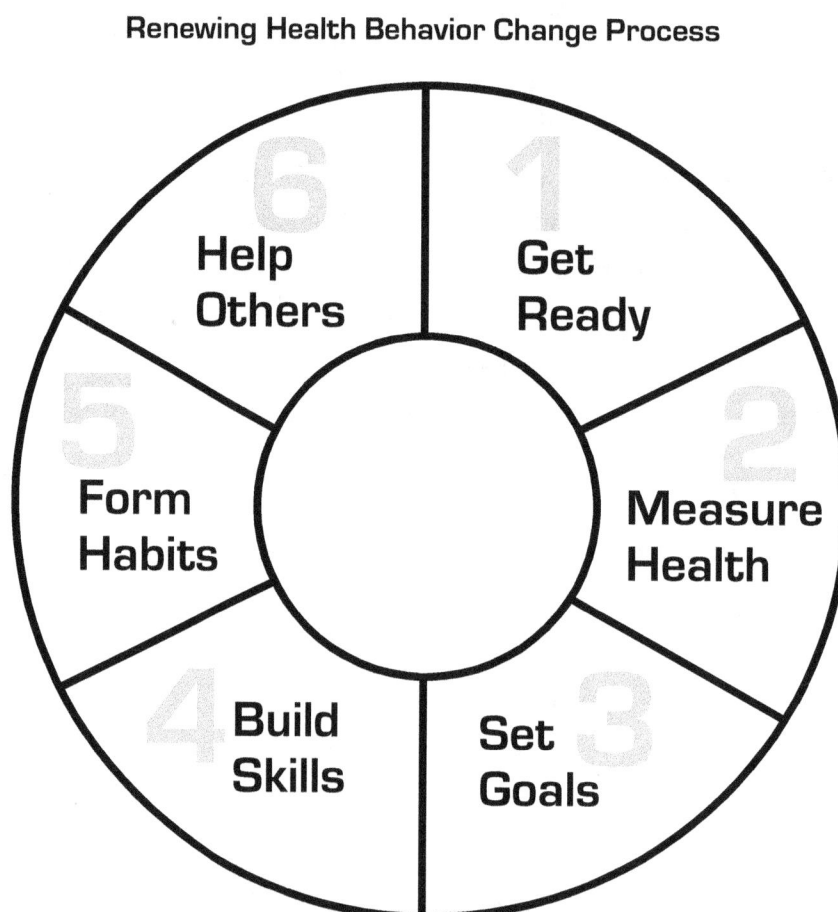

Step 1. Get Ready. Getting ready is about opening your heart and mind to change. It is about imagining what might become of your life. It is about reflecting on what is most important to you in life and starting to think about health relative to other priorities. This is also a time to reflect on how better health can help you realize your passions. Asking people to open their minds in this way can reduce some of the resistance people often feel about making any type of change in life. This step can be part of the process that moves people from the precontemplation to the contemplation stage of *readiness to change*.[10] The critical element of this step is empowering people to dream about what might be and helping them believe they control their own destiny.

·   A health promotion program can support the Get Ready step through multi-media promotional campaigns and interactive discussions.

Step 2. Measure Your Health. People who open their hearts and minds to change will be eager to measure their health. In the context of a health promotion program, the best measures of health are a health risk appraisal (HRA) and a basic health screening. Biometric measures included in screenings evolve over time, but the most common currently are blood pressure and resting heart rate; blood glucose, triglycerides and cholesterol (total, HDL, LDL and LDL/HDL ratio); and height, weight, waist and hip measurements. Collectively, these tests measure metabolic syndrome, which is the likelihood a person will contract diabetes, stroke or heart disease sometime in the future.[11] If a person has abnormal values in three of the five areas, they have metabolic syndrome.

Most HRAs focus on the physical dimensions of health and some examine the social or cultural dimensions. To measure the emotional, social and spiritual dimensions, free questionnaires offered by The Soul/Body Connection can be used. These questionnaires measure hope, humor, optimism, spirituality and well-being, forgiveness and gratitude (http://www.spiritualityhealth.com). Measures developed by the Authentic Happiness group assess core strengths, emotions, engagement, meaning and life satisfaction (http://www.authentichappiness.sas.upenn.edu/). Another valuable supplement is the Physical Activity Readiness Questionnaire (PAR-Q) developed by the Expert Advisory Committee of the Canadian Society for Exercise Physiology and the British Columbia Ministry of Health (http://uwfitness.uwaterloo.ca/PDF/par-q.pdf). This is a good tool to identify physical conditions that require a physician's clearance before an exercise program.

· A health promotion program can support the Measure Your Health step by offering a health risk appraisal and health screening programs.

Step 3. Set Goals. Setting goals is important to success in any area of life. If you don't know what you want, how do you know the first step to take to get there? How do you know if you are making good progress? Setting goals is also one of the most important things you can do to improve your health. In fact, a review by Goetzel and Heaney[12] concluded that personal goal setting can double success rates in health promotion programs. Goal setting is part science and part art, but there is more science than most people think. Both are briefly summarized below.

Impact of setting goals. Setting goals, especially challenging goals, increases performance in many ways. Setting goals helps us focus our attention on activities that will lead

The face of Wellness
A Conceptual Framework to Guide the Development of Effective Health Promotion Programs:
The Awareness, Motivation, Skills and Opportunity (AMSO) Framework and The Face of Wellness Model

to achieving these goals.[13] Setting goals also increases the physical effort we are willing to exert when we get fatigued, and helps us tolerate repetitive tasks that lead to our goal.[14] Setting goals also helps us prolong effort,[15] and stimulates us to draw on our knowledge to develop strategies to meet our goals.[16]

Types of goals. There are three types of goals and different strategies are recommended for each type.[17] The goal types are aspirational, learning and performance. Aspirational goals are dreams about what the future may be. These might include career ambitions, romantic relationships, raising a family, athletic performance, a specific body image, a sense of confidence, living a life of integrity, or other dreams. Aspirational goals do not need to be realistic, specific or static. They should be about dreams, about what makes you feel fulfilled, about priorities in life. They often evolve as life evolves. Learning goals can be tied to gaining specific knowledge necessary to achieve an aspirational goal, but people tend to be more committed to learning and actually learn more, when they allow themselves some latitude to explore what interests them. This is especially true in areas that are complex or novel to them.[18] Once a person has acquired the knowledge and ability to perform specific tasks, setting specific goals leads to higher performance.[19] For example, the aspirational goal might be to get rid of all the junk food in your diet and replace it with nutritious food. The learning goal might be to learn how to identify, shop for and prepare delicious nutritious foods. Once the knowledge and skills are acquired, the performance goal might be to eat nutritious foods at least 90% of the time.

Challenging goals. Once skills and knowledge are acquired, setting specific performance goals increases performance by 42%-82%, while setting challenging goals tends to increase performance or effort by 52%-82%.[20] These results are likely to occur only when commitment to the performance goal is high, and the person possesses the necessary skills and the ability to achieve the goal. For example, it is realistic to set specific and ambitious goals related to performing specific amounts and types of exercises or activities, and eating specific amounts and types of food because these are behaviors that are under a person's control. It is not realistic to set a specific and ambitious weight loss goal, because losing weight is a condition, not a distinct behavior that is within a person's total control.

Setting your own goals. Setting your own goals rather than relying on an expert or advisor can increase performance by 11%[21], probably because people tend to better understand goals they set for themselves.[22] Nonetheless, skilled advisors can be very helpful in setting goals.

Commitment. Goal performance is strongest when commitment to goals is strongest. Commitment can be enhanced by reinforcing the importance of the outcome and by enhancing self efficacy. Commitment can also be increased by making a public commitment to the goal,[23] and by receiving support from leaders. [24] Self-efficacy can be enhanced by providing adequate training to increase mastery, observing positive role models, and hearing persuasive communication from experts or peers who express confidence in your ability to achieve the goal.[25]

Feedback. Regular feedback also enhances performance. When people realize they are falling short of their goals, they normally increase their effort or shift to a more effective strategy.[26]

In summary, goal setting will be most effective when five processes are followed:

1. Allow aspirational goals to evolve over time.

2. Allow some latitude in setting learning goals to acquire the skills and knowledge necessary to tackle a goal.

3. Set challenging and specific performance goals with input from experts if possible. Include short term and intermediate measurable milestone targets. Limit performance goals to activities that are under your control.

4. Seek feedback and monitor progress. Increase effort or modify strategies if goals are not being met.

5. Enhance commitment through public statements of commitment and inspiring comments from leaders.

    ·   A health promotion program can support the *Set Goals* step by offering goal setting sessions in group, print and web format. Aspirational goals typically begin to emerge during the initial *Get Ready* step. Learning and performance goals take form during the *Build Skills* step.

The face of Wellness
A Conceptual Framework to Guide the Development of Effective Health Promotion Programs:
The Awareness, Motivation, Skills and Opportunity (AMSO) Framework and The Face of Wellness Model

Step 4. Build Skills. If you were going to learn a new language, what would you do? The best strategy would be to immerse yourself in a culture that speaks that language, so you could hear people speak, watch how their lips and face move as they express each of the words and phrases, learn about their customs so you could better understand the underlying meaning of phrases. You would also need to learn grammar rules and vocabulary. Using books, tapes or a language coach might help you. You would also need to practice, practice, practice. If you were going to learn how to play soccer, you could start by watching others play. You would need to learn the rules by reading manuals and talking to people. At some point you would need to meet people who play soccer so you could play with them. To get good, you need to learn the individual moves, how to dribble with your feet, how to trap (or catch) a ball with your feet or any other part of your body (except your hands), how to pass or take a shot on goal. If you want to get really good, you need to learn how to dribble past a defender with speed or finesse, how to kick a ball that is six feet off the ground by doing a modified back flip, or put spin on the ball when you kick it, so it changes direction in mid air to go over or around a defender. Having the right books, a coach, and patient teammates really helps during this process. Eventually, you need to internalize the rules, know the rules without thinking, so you don't go off-sides, commit a foul, or get yourself thrown out of the game. To play at the highest level, you need to master the individual moves so you perform them instinctually when an opportunity presents itself. You also need to learn mental toughness so you can keep playing full speed when you are exhausted, hurt, or way behind.

Changing a health behavior is a lot like learning a new language or playing a new sport, except it is usually a lot harder, because you need to break habits you have formed over decades of time. If you could immerse yourself in a culture that supports your new lifestyle, it would be a lot easier, but that is not an option for most people. So you have to find or build subcultures that can support you, and teach you how to resist the influences of the cultures that have supported the unhealthy habits you have learned and practiced for decades. Think about it. You have indeed honed those old habits through decades of practice, practice, practice. They are part of you. You perform them without thinking. They are comfortable. They are part of your identity. You need to learn new habits, and learning new habits usually takes months and often takes years. In the case of quitting smoking or chewing tobacco, you also have to overcome a chemical addiction to nicotine. Weight loss is even more complicated because you cannot just quit eating. You must learn how to eat differently. If you are going to be successful in changing your health habits, you need to build new skills.

The skill building process has three basic stages: learning, practicing and building support. Celebrating progress in moving through these stages reinforces each of them. The stages are described in more detail below.

Learning. One of the first steps in learning is figuring out how you like to learn and how much help you need. The key is to match the complexity of the change you want to make with the amount and form of help you draw upon. If you want to change something simple, like starting to floss your teeth every night, you can probably get a brochure from your dentist or simple instructions on the web. If you want to lose 100 pounds, you need more help. Individually directed options include reading, listening to tapes, or following web-based programs. Expert-directed options include working with a counselor or coach through individual or group sessions on the telephone or face-to-face. People are more likely to stick with learning formats suited to their learning style and schedule. Most people benefit from some direct interaction with a real person, even if most of their learning is self-directed. Utilizing the most scientifically validated strategies can have tremendous benefit. For example, people who try to quit smoking cold turkey are successful about 5% of the time, while those who use a combination of behavioral therapy and medication are successful about 30% of the time.[27]

Practicing. The simple act of practicing a new behavior is an important step in building confidence that you can perform the behavior. This is called enhancing self-efficacy.[28] The higher the level of self-efficacy, the longer the newly acquired behavior will be practiced before relapse.

Building support and reinforcement. Most people are successful in continuing a behavior if they have access to a physical environment that makes that behavior easy to perform, and a network of people to encourage them. Making sure these pieces are in place during the skill building stage can increase the chances of maintaining these new behaviors long term. For example, if you want to exercise on a regular bases, you need a place to do it. Some people can be successful walking or running in their neighborhoods and doing calisthenics without equipment. Other people need the equipment provided by a fitness center. Similarly, some people can maintain their programs on their own but most people benefit from having a network of friends to join them in workouts. The same concepts apply to all health behaviors. For example, to eat a nutritious diet, you need to have access to grocery stores and cafeterias that sell the right food. If you live with other people, they need to at least tolerate the foods you choose to eat.

The face of Wellness
A Conceptual Framework to Guide the Development of Effective Health Promotion Programs:
The Awareness, Motivation, Skills and Opportunity (AMSO) Framework and The Face of Wellness Model

Celebrating Progress. Recognizing and celebrating milestones is very reinforcing for many people. Milestones might include (1) making a commitment to change; (2) developing a change plan; (3) learning the skills you need to change; (4) trying out each new skill for the first time; (5) practicing each new skill on a regular basis; (6) achieving performance goals – for example, exercising for 30 minutes, three times a week for a full week; and (7) making incremental progress in achieving an aspirational goal (i.e., losing a certain number of pounds, reaching different strength levels, etc.). For many people, just pausing to reflect on the effort you have exerted to reach this goal, and realizing you have achieved it, is a sufficient celebration. Many people like to include some more significant celebrations. The key is to choose celebrations that you value, support your wellness goal and are healthy for you in general. Many cultures around the world equate celebration with splurging on food... usually high fat, sweet food, or drinking lots of alcohol. Why not? Its fun and it feels great... at first. It also leads to all the health problems discussed in this workbook. Splurging on food might not be a great way to celebrate your wellness milestones, especially if you are trying to loose weight. Working through each of these issues during the Build Skills stage increases the chances of maintaining long-term behavior change.

> · A health promotion program can support the *Build Skills* step by offering skill building programs for each of the health change areas (fitness, nutrition, stress management, weight control, quit smoking, etc.) in multiple learning formats (i.e., print, web, telephonic, video, face to face, etc.)

Step 5. Form Habits. Dieting doesn't work. Virtually everyone who goes on a diet to lose weight fails. They fail not because they don't lose weight. In fact, most well-conceived diets do produce weight loss...for a few weeks or months. Diets usually fail because most people revert to their old eating habits when they reach their weight goal...and they regain their weight. People succeed in losing weight and keeping it off when they change how they eat... forever. The same is true for getting fit. Working out for a month or a year gets you in shape for that month or year, but when you stop exercising, you eventually get out of shape. The key to successful long-term health behavior change is to build your newly formed health skills into habits you practice every single week, and in most cases, every single day.

When you add a new positive behavior to your life, it often takes months of diligent discipline to keep practicing the new behavior. An addictive behavior, like smoking cigarettes, can take as much as 5 to 12 years of diligent discipline to change permanently. Most of the time you feel the immediate rewards of your new behavior, and that keeps you going, but remaining disciplined is draining work for most people. If you can build the new behavior into your routine, you take away the need to discipline yourself.

Your routines change over the span of a lifetime, and you need to adapt with these changes in routines to form new habits around exercise. A high school student involved in sports works out during varsity sports practices. Going to practice becomes the habit. A college student enrolled in gym classes is physically active during those classes. The changing schedule of classes does not matter because the habit formed becomes taking a gym class. An adult involved in a team sport forms the habit of going to team practice. Over time, getting a regular workout becomes one of the important ingredients in a successful day and is squeezed in regardless of the challenges.

- Health promotion programs can support the *Form Habits* step through programming, community networks, policy changes and enhancing the physical environment. Programming options include offering ongoing classes on nutritious cooking, aerobics, yoga, ballroom dancing, and other types of physical activity and support groups for people who have quit smoking or lost weight. Community networks can include sports teams and leagues, discounts negotiated with local fitness centers, and improved access to fresh produce markets. Physical environment supports can include cafeterias that serve nutritious foods, work sites built to make stairs more accessible than elevators and floor plans that encourage other forms of walking. Policy supports can include smoke free policies, health insurance coverage of health promotion services, and many other options.

Step 6. Help Others. The final step in the Renewing Health Behavior Change Process is helping others. Helping others can take the form of serving as a peer mentor, organizing or leading a support group or an activity group, learning how to teach a skill building course, serving on a planning committee, helping to promote a program, or many other forms. Helping others has at least four benefits.

First, it reinforces a newly adopted behavior. Everything you learn to help yourself become a leader can help you learn how to maintain the new behavior in your own life. Additionally, knowing that other people are depending on you makes you want to serve as a good role model for the new behavior and reinforces your commitment to that behavior.

The face of Wellness
A Conceptual Framework to Guide the Development of Effective Health Promotion Programs:
The Awareness, Motivation, Skills and Opportunity (AMSO) Framework and The Face of Wellness Model

Second, helping others provides an inspiration for others to change. When people see that someone else has been successful in changing their behavior and has progressed beyond that to helping other people, it increases their belief they can be successful in making the same kind of change.

Third, helping other people seems to have a direct protective effect on health, especially for older adults.[29] Helping others also allows people to show compassion, which seems to have a direct positive impact on health.

Finally, as more and more people extend themselves to help others, more people can be helped.

· Health promotion programs can support the *Help Others* stage by making it very clear that peer leaders are critical to the success of the program, carving out defined leadership opportunities, training people how to serve in these roles, and thanking them for the contributions they make.

Ongoing Renewal

Helping Others is listed as the sixth and final step in the Renewing Health Behavior Change Process but there is really no final step. The Process is illustrated in a circle, because it is really an ongoing process. When you are successful in achieving one health behavior change, this is a good time to reflect on progress, celebrate success, renew commitment to that change, take a deep breath, and ask yourself if you are ready to tackle another health behavior change. The satisfaction and self-confidence that comes from feeling successful in making the first change will often propel you through the difficult early stages of the next change. Other great times to reflect on health and get ready to make another change are anniversary dates and the beginning of the new year.

· A health promotion program can support the overall Renewing Health Behavior Change Process by making the steps in the process clear, encouraging people to move through each of the six steps, and providing tools to help people document and celebrate their progress through the steps.

Awareness, Motivation, Skills and Opportunities

In 1984[30], I suggested that we think of health promotion programs in terms of three components: Awareness, Behavior Change and Supportive Environments. In 2005, I started advocating that we shift the paradigm to think in terms of four areas: Awareness, Motivation, Skills and Opportunity [AMSO], i.e. the AMSO Framework.[31] The purpose of this change in terminology is to shift the focus of health promotion from the work of health promotion providers to the experiences of the people and organizations served. The AMSO Framework is illustrated in the form of a triangle to evoke the image commonly used to describe how money should be allocated in different investment vehicles in an investment portfolio. Within the facial image of the Face of Wellness Model, the AMSO Framework represents the nose [Figure 5].

Figure 5

**Portfolio Balancing Approach to Planning Change Strategies:
Awareness, Motivation, Skills and Opportunity**

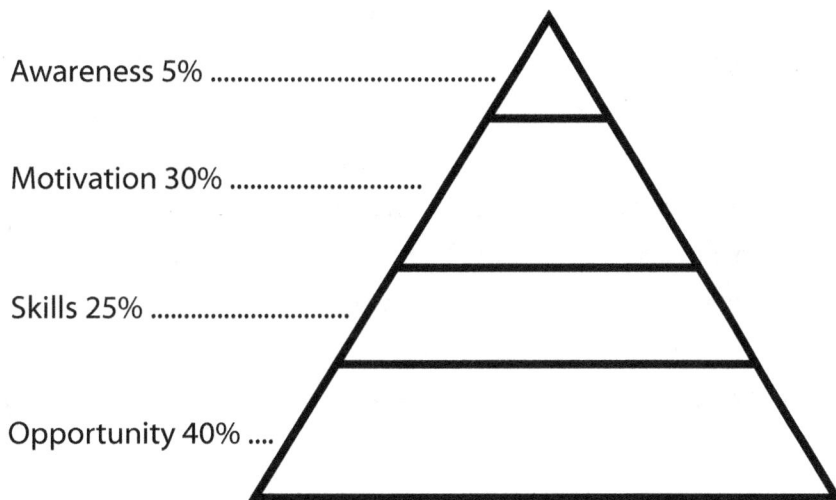

Awareness 5%

Motivation 30%

Skills 25%

Opportunity 40%

Awareness

The origins of health promotion are in health education, and as the term implies, health education focuses on making people aware of the risks of unhealthy behaviors such as eating

The face of Wellness
A Conceptual Framework to Guide the Development of Effective Health Promotion Programs:
The Awareness, Motivation, Skills and Opportunity (AMSO) Framework and The Face of Wellness Model

an unhealthy diet, drinking excessively and smoking, as well as the benefits of positive behaviors such as regular health screenings, physical activity and stress management. Our belief was that people would make the right choices if they just had the right information, i.e. the right education. Most health promotion programs in the 1970s and 1980s were based on an educational model, and many still are. Over time, we have learned that education is not enough to change behavior for most people. Most people know that they SHOULD exercise. Most smokers know that smoking causes many forms of cancer, respiratory problems, and heart disease, and that it is likely to contribute to their early demise. If knowledge were enough, no one would smoke and everyone would exercise.

This is not to say that education is not important. Education plays at least two important roles. First, effective education campaigns do make people aware of health risks and health improvement opportunities. For people who are considering making a behavior change, education can help them weigh the pros and cons of making the change, and lead them to the resources they need to support their change efforts. Second, education campaigns can be critical in mobilizing organization- or nation-wide change efforts in building broad support for an idea or plan. For example, when people realized that secondhand smoke is not just irritating, but a Class A carcinogen, efforts to create smoke-free workplaces were perceived as strategies to protect workers instead of strategies to punish smokers. Despite the limited impact of education on behavior change, it is still important to improve the effectiveness of education efforts, and excellent progress has been made in this area. Improvements have included learning how to tailor messages to address people's individual needs, providing multiple formats in which to convey content (lecture, print, audiotape, Internet, e-mail, etc.), and harnessing data management and communication capabilities to store, manage, retrieve, and deliver data. Despite these developments, education simply is not enough to change behavior for most people, and managers need to realize this in designing and evaluating programs.

Motivation

When a person is motivated to make a behavior change, s/he will strive to gain the know-ledge and skills necessary to make that change, and will create the opportunity to make it possible. If a person is not motivated to change, all the knowledge and skills in the world will still not cause change. For example, testing of the Theory of Planned Behavior[32] developed by Fishbien and Aizen has shown that attitudes and norms have little effect on behavior unless a person has intentions to change. Knowledge of the importance of motivation and measuring motivation has improved substantially in the past few decades. One of the most important developments in this area has been articulation of the concept of motivational readiness to change, as articulated in the **Transtheoretical Model** by Prochaska and DiClemente.[33] This model shows us that different strategies are important to motivate people to change at different levels of readiness to change. For example, it shows us that people who are not thinking about change in the near future (precontemplation) have no interest in hearing about how to change their behavior, but those thinking about changes (contemplation) might be interested in this information. It also shows us that enhancing self-efficacy is important to those getting ready to make changes (preparation), those in the process of making changes (action), and those who are working to maintain changes (maintenance).

Progress has also been made in explaining how *intrinsic* and *extrinsic incentives* motivate people to join programs and change behaviors. For example, a review by Matson-Koffman et al.[34] showed that financial incentives have the impact of significantly increasing participation rates. This probably occurs because incentives capture the attention of people who are thinking about making changes (contemplators) and accelerates their decision to make a change, and possibly even those not thinking about making a change (precontemplators) because they are attracted by the money. Matson's review also showed that financial incentive programs do not increase behavior change success rates in most cases. This is not surprising for two reasons. First, if incentives attract people who are less committed to making a change into programs, we would expect fewer of those people to succeed. Second, financial incentive programs are based on the assumption that money is important to everyone. To a certain extent, this is true. To those with modest incomes, a few hundred dollars can make a big difference in helping to meet basic needs in any given week or month, but over the course of a year, this translates to only a few dollars a week, and will not make much difference in any budget. Millions of people with limited incomes find a way to spend $20 to $100 dollars a week, or $1000 to $5000 a year, on cigarettes. If money were a sufficient motivator, no one would smoke. For a wealthy person, a financial incentive of a few hundred dollars is little more than a pleasant gift; it makes no impact on other spending decisions. To be effective in producing significant change, a financial reward would need to be large enough to impact someone's financial well-being, and this is just not feasible for most health promotion programs.

The prevalence of financial incentives in workplace health promotion programs is likely to increase significantly over the next decade because of Section 2705 of the Affordable Care Act passed in 2010. Section 2705 confirmed in statute what had previously been articulated only

The face of Wellness
A Conceptual Framework to Guide the Development of Effective Health Promotion Programs:
The Awareness, Motivation, Skills and Opportunity (AMSO) Framework and The Face of Wellness Model

in federal regulations, i.e. that employers are permitted to offer a differential in health plan premiums of up to 20% for employees who meet health standards compared to employees who do not. These standards can be set by employers, but typically include choosing to participate in a program, not smoking, having a recommended weight, and having normal biometrics. The maximum premium differential is scheduled to increase to 30% in 2014 and the Secretaries of Treasury and Health and Human Services were given authority to increase the amount to 50% in 2014. Given the findings of a growing body of research,[35] implementation of these policies is likely to significantly increase participation in health promotion programs. For example, Seaverson et al[36] found that participation rates in health risk assessments were in the 20% - 40% range for workplace programs that had strong leadership support and well designed marketing programs and 70% to 90% and higher for programs that also offered financial incentives. The 90% and higher participation rates were achieved by employers who provided a financial incentive by reducing the amount of the health plan premium or deductible. Employer adoption of these programs took a big jump as soon as the Affordable Care Act passed. According to a survey of large employers in 2009, 36% offered financial incentives for participating in programs and 8% for achieving health goals in 2009. By 2012, those values jumped to 80% for participation and 38% for health outcomes.[37]

Despite the effectiveness of financial incentives in motivating people to participate in programs, we should not over rely on financial or other extrinsic incentives. The biggest shortcomings in our efforts to motivate people have been our focus on extrinsic rewards such as money and gifts, which capture short-term attention, rather than intrinsic rewards that are part of a person's basic values. If we want to be effective in motivating people, we need to first understand their passions in life, long-term goals, and current priorities. For example, I spent a year in Seoul, Korea, as a visiting professor in the department of preventive medicine of a university. Although most of the faculty in my department did not smoke, the smoking rate among physician professors in departments of preventive medicine in Korea as a whole was close to the smoking rate of men in general, which was over 60%. Lack of knowledge of the health risks of smoking was clearly not the issue with these physicians; I quickly learned that discussions of the health risks of smoking were fruitless. After a few months of observing the culture, I realized the importance within the Korean culture of being a good role model, especially among physician educators. When I asked my smoking colleagues about the message their smoking behavior was sending to their medical students, their patients, and their own children, they were far more receptive to thinking about quitting. Discussing smoking in this context shifted them from precontemplation to contemplation.

This strategy could probably work with anyone. For example, I once met an older woman who was sedentary and overweight. She had no interest in exercise and had become content with the belief that she always had been and always would be overweight. The priority in her life was spending time with her grandchildren. When she realized that playing with her grandchildren for a few hours exhausted her, and that she might not live long enough to attend her granddaughter's wedding, she decided to start a regular exercise program . . . in the form of playing with her grandchildren. Another example: A friend in college started smoking when he was in high school and continued smoking when he went to college. He was strong and energetic and felt impervious to any health risks smoking might cause in twenty years or thirty years. He did not stop smoking until he got a serious crush on a beautiful young woman. She made him leave the room whenever he smoked, her feelings were hurt when he said the food she cooked for him was bland, and she hated kissing him because his mouth smelled so bad. He decided to quit smoking because he thought he would lose her. He was sure he had made the right decision when he realized how much money he was saving and now had available to take her out on dates. These examples illustrate that improving health is often not the motivation for many behavior changes, even though most health professionals think improving health is a primary motivator. If we are to be successful in helping people change their health behaviors, we must understand their passions, long-term goals, and current priorities. The process of Motivational Interviewing developed by Miller and Rolnick[38] provides an excellent framework for this process. Some health promotion professionals are beginning to apply this important process in their programming efforts. Describing optimal health in terms of the five dimensions of optimal health, and encouraging each individual to put their passions in the heart of their programs is also likely to engage many people. The challenge, of course, is the high cost of taking the time to do this on a one-to-one basis. It may be possible to develop computer-based strategies for this work. Some health promotion providers have developed online tailoring programs that do much of this.

Enhancing self-efficacy is another way to enhance motivation.[25] **Self-efficacy** is the belief that one can do something, like exercise regularly, quit smoking, give a speech, etc. **Behavioral efficacy** is the belief that a specific behavior will produce a specific outcome – for example, that quitting smoking will reduce the likelihood of developing lung cancer. The higher the level of self-efficacy and the behavioral efficacy, the greater the motivation.

Our overall understanding of how to motivate people in the context of a health promotion program is probably the biggest gap in our health promotion knowledge. If we can fill this gap, we are likely to see the participation and success rates soar.

The face of Wellness
A Conceptual Framework to Guide the Development of Effective Health Promotion Programs:
The Awareness, Motivation, Skills and Opportunity (AMSO) Framework and The Face of Wellness Model

Skills

The biggest shortcoming of awareness programs is that they tell people WHAT to do, but not HOW to do it. Skill-building programs show people HOW—how to perform the actual behaviors they should perform, how to integrate these behaviors into their lives, and how to change their environment and surroundings to create opportunities to practice the behaviors they need to practice. Skill building strategies are discussed above as the third step of the individual Renewing Health Behavior Change Process.

Opportunity

Earlier editions of this workbook[30,39,40] articulated the concept of a supportive environment as one that includes supportive culture, policies, facilities, and programming. Given the goal discussed earlier of shifting the focus of the work of health promotion professionals from an internal focus on the work they do to the perspective of the people they serve, this edition uses the broader concept of opportunity.

Having access to opportunities to practice a healthy lifestyle is one of the most important factors in helping a person advance from building new skills (step 4 above) to forming habits (step 5 above).

A person who is highly motivated to practice a healthy lifestyle and has well-developed skills to integrate these practices into his or her life can do a lot to create the opportunities necessary to make this a reality. However, sometimes a person's life situation is so de-manding, or his or her physical surroundings so limited, that creating the necessary op-portunities is very difficult, even for a highly motivated and skilled person. Most people are only moderately motivated and moderately skilled and need even more support to make a behavior change. They need convenient access to affordable, delicious, nutritious foods; safe and fun places to be physically active; smoke-free air to breathe at home, work, and play; exposure to supportive friends and family, and to a culture that values and rewards good health; freedom from media, advertising, and other marketing influences that are peddling risky behaviors; time to devote to healthy endeavors that are difficult to integrate into daily routines; and sufficient protection from the stresses of finances, overly demanding work, abusive social situations, and safety threats to be able to focus on good health practices.

At the other extreme, an abundantly supportive environment can cause an unmotivated, unskilled person to practice very healthy habits. At a health spa, it's easy to eat delicious, low-calorie, nutritious food at every meal, because that is all that is served. It is easy to go for a swim when you wake up, go for a long hike before lunch, do yoga before a late afternoon nap, and take time to reflect on the priorities of life in the evening. There are talented and charming experts to guide you, interesting, motivated people to join you, and all the time you need to do whatever you want. The biggest shortcoming of a spa experience is that the wonderful supports that make it easy to practice a healthy lifestyle stay at the spa when you leave. For some people, the experience of eating well, exercising regularly, and relaxing in a spa setting shows them that it is possible to do these things, and gives them a sense of the physical and emotional rewards these things provide. This enhances their self-efficacy and behavioral efficacy. This sense of enhanced self-efficacy and behavioral efficacy increases motivation to continue performing these behaviors. If the spa can also teach people the skills to integrate the new behaviors into their lives and continue them as part of a normal life, successful maintenance is much more likely. The other great shortcoming of a spa situation is that most people do not have the financial resources to spend the $1000-per-day or higher fees charged by the best spas. It is possible to create supportive environments in any workplace or community setting if there is sufficient will. The cost is on the order of $200 to $400 per person per year for a comprehensive program, including the awareness, skill-building, motivational, and supportive environment components. In a workplace setting, supportive environments will include physical environments, organizational policies, organizational culture, and ongoing programs and structures that encourage healthy lifestyle, and strategies to ensure that employees feel a sense of ownership for the program [Table 4]. Workplace health promotion programs have so much potential to improve the health of employees because employees spend a large portion of their waking hours at work, usually over a long span of time. They develop close long-term relationships with work colleagues and can be influenced in positive ways by the organizational culture. However, employees are exposed to many influences beyond the workplace that create an abundance of opportunities to develop positive or negative health habits. Health promotion programs will have the greatest successes if they account for all these many influences and opportunities.

The face of Wellness
A Conceptual Framework to Guide the Development of Effective Health Promotion Programs:
The Awareness, Motivation, Skills and Opportunity (AMSO) Framework and The Face of Wellness Model

Table 4

Elements of a Supportive Environment

Physical Environments

Healthy food in cafeteria

Smoke-free environment

Ergonomically sound furniture

Protection from injury hazards

Opportunities to be physically active

Organization Policies

Medical coverage of preventive services

Consumer-driven health plan

Absenteeism policy that rewards being healthy

Smoke-free environment

Flexible benefits and flextime

Management policies that moderate stress

Organization Culture

Healthy role models

Incentive systems

Communication systems

Peer support

Table 4 continued

Ongoing Programs and Structures
· ·

Health promotion department

Coaching and mentoring

Employee assistance programs

Child care programs

Recreation programs

Employee Ownership and Involvement
· ·

Program design

Program promotion

Program delivery

Program leadership

Program evaluation

The face of Wellness
A Conceptual Framework to Guide the Development of Effective Health Promotion Programs:
The Awareness, Motivation, Skills and Opportunity (AMSO) Framework and The Face of Wellness Model

POSSE[2]: The Dimensions of Opportunity

POSSE[2] is a pneumonic device created to organize a vast range of factors that influence the opportunities a person is able to access. Posse is defined as "*a large group with a common interest*" by the Merriam Webster Dictionary,[41] and as "*your crew, your homies, people who sometimes have your back*" by the Urban Dictionary.[42] The six components of POSSE[2] are listed and discussed below.

P: Peers

O: Organizations

S: State

S: Society

E: Environment

E: Equality

P: Peers

The health behaviors and attitudes of close friends and co-workers, especially people we consider our peers, have a significant impact on our health habits. This is clearly illustrated in a series of studies conducted by Nicholas Christakis, James Fowler and colleagues on the impact of the health habits of friends, family members, and neighbors on each other, drawing from data in the Framingham Heart Study.[43] The Framingham study involved 12,067 people spanning three generations, with longitudinal data on health habits and health outcomes collected eight times between 1973 and 2003. As shown in figure 6, an individual is nearly 175% more likely to become obese if a close friend (referred to as "mutual" friend in the figure) becomes obese. As the strength of the emotional connection to the person becoming obese decreases, the association also decreases. For example, the individual is 50%-75% more likely to become obese when a same sex friend, a same sex sibling or ego-perceived friend (someone you consider a friend but they do not consider you a friend) becomes obese. The likelihood of becoming obese does not increase substantially or at all when an opposite-sex friend, an immediate neighbor, or an alter-perceived friend (someone who considers you a friend but you do not consider a friend) becomes obese.[44] This team found similar but less pronounced patterns for tobacco use,[45] depression,[46] and alcohol use.[47]

Figure 6

Probability of Becoming Obese if Others Become Obese

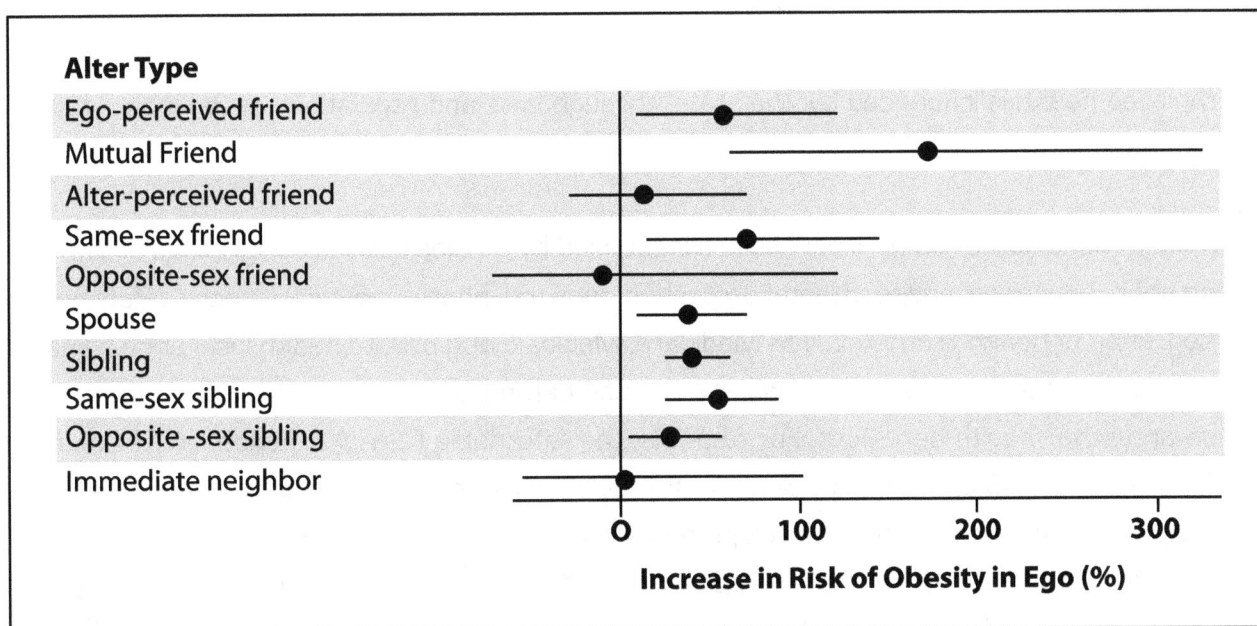

Chrisakis NA, Fowler JH.N Engl J Med.2007; 357; 370-379.

O: Organizations

Employers have a tremendous influence on the health habits of their workforces. Channels of influence include the formal health promotion programs they offer, access to fitness centers and other places to be physically active, nutritious food served in cafeterias, protection from exposure to toxic substances including second hand tobacco smoke, policies related to absenteeism, medical insurance, and environmental sustainability as well as the management style of leaders and the core values and mission of the organization.

The face of Wellness
A Conceptual Framework to Guide the Development of Effective Health Promotion Programs:
The Awareness, Motivation, Skills and Opportunity (AMSO) Framework and The Face of Wellness Model

Despite the magnitude of its influence, employers represent just one of the organizations that influence people's health habits. For families with children, schools, child care centers, entertainment outlets, grocery stores and restaurants all have a powerful influence. For families of faith, churches, synagogues, mosques and other religious centers shape priorities in life, increase access to services and influence health choices in other ways. Social clubs, professional networks, food and entertainment outlets all influence people's attitudes and perceptions as well as their access to programs and services. Employers need to learn how to leverage these influences, or overcome them, to be successful in enhancing the health of their employees.

S: State

Employee health is influenced by "the state" through laws and regulations at the local, state and national level.

At the national level, health practices are influenced by policies related to agriculture, transportation, education, environmental protection, tobacco, pharmaceuticals, social safety net, integration of health promotion into Medicare, Medicaid and private health insurance plans, support for medical research as well as specific campaigns on fitness, nutrition, tobacco use and other health behaviors. For example, the Affordable Care Act passed in March of 2011 included 38 specific provisions that integrate health promotion into national health policy. These provisions include development of an annual National Prevention Strategy, providing grants to help small employers develop health promotion programs, allowing employers to provide reduced health plan premiums to employees who meet health goals, providing reimbursement for Medicare beneficiaries to have an annual wellness exam and access to lifestyle change programs, testing the impact of health promotion programs on health and costs for Medicaid recipients and many other provisions.[48]

At the state level, important policies include gun safety, road speed limits, motorcycle helmet rules, Medicaid eligibility and scope of services covered, pollution protection and tobacco policy support. For example, there is significant variation by state in requiring smoke free workplaces and public places, amounts of state taxes charged on tobacco sales, support for tobacco prevention and cessation efforts, allowing employers to set their own policies about hiring smokers, and the portion of the tobacco Master Settlement Agreement (MSA) devoted to tobacco prevention and cessation efforts. For example, the Centers for Disease Control and Prevention (CDC) developed recommendations for how much each state should spend on state tobacco prevention programs based the size of its population, the amount it receives annually from the MSA, and the cost and effectiveness of various tobacco prevention and treatment strategies. In 2012, Alaska ranked 1st (best) spending $10.8 million, 101% of the 10.7 million recommended by CDC. Ohio tied for 50th (worst) with Missouri, Connecticut, District of Columbia, Nevada, and New Hampshire, spending $0 on these programs. Under Governor John Kasich, Ohio became the only state in the nation that did not provide support to allow its residents to access the national 1-800-QUITNOW telephone quit line.[49] Earlier, in 2008, under the leadership of then Governor Ted Strickland, the Ohio legislature dismantled the Ohio Tobacco Prevention Foundation, one of the most effective state level tobacco prevention organizations ever created, and used the funding to support the Governor's budget priorities.[50] Declines in the smoking rate leveled off shortly after these policy changes were implemented.

Local policies include zoning laws allowing mixed use real estate developments, active transportation options and construction of sidewalks, bike paths and pedestrian malls, prohibition of use of toxic ingredients in restaurants, smoke-free work and public place policies, excise taxes on tobacco, protection from pollution and outreach campaigns in each of the healthy lifestyle areas. Policies in New York City are probably the most effective in the nation in terms of promoting healthy lifestyle.[51]

Employers have the choice of being passive or active citizens in establishing local and state health policies, and to some extent in national health policies. For example, under the leadership of CEO Dr. Toby Cosgrove, the Cleveland Clinic decided to become very active in state and local tobacco policy. They established smoke-free campuses at their nearly 100 hospital and clinic locations in 2005, developed an intensive tobacco treatment program for patients, helped pass a state law establishing smoke-free policies in all work and public places and helped pass a county law increasing excise tax on cigarettes in 2006, provided free nicotine replacement therapy (NRT) for all residents in Cuyahoga County (county in which most Cleveland Clinic hospitals and clinics are located) who called the state quitline (1-800-QUITNOW) in 2007, and stopped hiring smokers in 2008. Collectively, these policies drove smoking rates in Cuyahoga County from 26% in 2003 to 15% in 2009. By way of comparison, rates dropped from 25% to 21% for the rest of the State of Ohio and 22% to 18% for the United States during the same time period. By getting involved in these state and local policy efforts, the Cleveland Clinic

The face of Wellness
A Conceptual Framework to Guide the Development of Effective Health Promotion Programs:
The Awareness, Motivation, Skills and Opportunity (AMSO) Framework and The Face of Wellness Model

was able to help its employees quit smoking and also to reinforce its image as a strong proponent of smoke-free living. These efforts to fight tobacco are consistent with the Cleveland Clinic's ongoing ranking as the #1 heart center in the nation.

S: Society

In addition to being strongly influenced by peers, people are also influenced by broad cultural norms of the society in which they live, ethnic norms of the people with whom they interact and celebrities prominent in the media.

Physical Activity. At the beginning of the running craze in the United States, running a marathon (26.2 miles) was considered the rare feat of highly developed athletes and an estimated 25,000 completed a marathon in 1976. Over the years, peoples' view of the marathon evolved to the point that people believed running a marathon was within the grasp of the average healthy person. In 2011, an estimated 518,000 finished a marathon.[52] Despite the fact that a large portion of the population remains sedentary, the portion of the population that is very active has increased substantially.

Tobacco Use. In the mid 1970s when the workplace health promotion field started to take hold in the United States, second-hand smoke was considered annoying by many non-smokers, but there were minimal restrictions on smoking in homes, restaurants, workplaces, even hospitals. Asking someone to not smoke, even in your own home, was considered to be rude. These norms have completely flipped; smoking is known to be deadly,[53] smoking is unusual in most work and entertainment settings, and smoking without asking is concerned rude in most settings. In fact, restrictions for entire states are very common. Comprehensive (workplace, restaurant, bars) smoke-free laws in effect increased from zero on December 31, 2000,[54] to 23 states by July 1, 2012. Furthermore, 29 states prohibit smoking in workplaces, 34 in restaurants, 29 in bars and 15 in casinos. An estimated 81% of the population of the United States is covered by smoke-free laws at the state or local level.[55] Not surprisingly, tobacco use is highest in the states that have the weakest smoking policies.[56]

Ethnic Norms. People's health habits are strongly influenced by ethnic and cultural norms in their families and communities related to expression of emotions, asking for help, and helping others, the significance of food, and the extent to with one's views should be imposed on others. For example, cultural value of familismo, respeto, simpatia and personalismo make Hispanic/Latino families want to protect their families from second hand smoke BUT also make them reluctant to ask neighbors to refrain from smoking.[57]

Celebrity Role Models. Celebrities have a significant impact on many people. For example, as Oprah Winfrey lost and gained weight over the past few decades, many people, especially women, have tracked and emulated her methods.[58] Similarly, the constant exposure of woman to the perfect bodies of starlets can lead some women, especially young women, to dissatisfaction with their own bodies and sometimes to eating disorders or excessive exercising.[59] Increased visibility of fit women can also have positive effects. For example, when Sushmita Sen became the first Indian women named Miss Universe in 1994, it stimulated a shift toward a positive view of fitness in the Indian culture, a culture that has historically favored spiritual and intellectual development over fitness.

For employers, the key is to be aware of the impact of these broad societal influences, harness them when possible, and be prepared to overcome them when necessary.

E: Environment

There is a growing body of evidence that the natural, built and policy environment has a significant impact on physical activity and eating habits, and an emerging literature showing that these habits can be improved by changing these environments. This field of inquiry was largely created by the Robert Wood Johnson Foundation through their programs in Active Living by Design,[60] Active Living Research[61] and more recently in Healthy Eating Research.[62] Growth is fastest in the active living research, with the number of research studies published growing from 30 in 2000 to 678 in 2010.

The basic idea of active living is that routine physical activity has been engineered out of many people's lives. In the 1950s and 1960s, most children walked to school every day. By the 1980s, most children took the bus or were driven. People used to live in complete neighborhoods that allowed them to walk to the store, to a movie or restaurant and sometimes to work. Today, many communities are so spread out that a car is necessary to go any place. Many communities are built for cars rather than pedestrians or bicycles. Rather than walk to the

The face of Wellness
A Conceptual Framework to Guide the Development of Effective Health Promotion Programs:
The Awareness, Motivation, Skills and Opportunity (AMSO) Framework and The Face of Wellness Model

corner for the bus or subway, people back out of their garages, drive to work and often park in the basement of the buildings where they work. Safety from crime is also a concern that keeps many people from walking, especially in poor neighborhoods. People use remote clickers to turn on the TV, send emails at work rather than walking down the hall and surf the net to do research rather than browse through the library. Many of these advances have significantly improved productivity, but they have also increased sedentary behaviors. One of the landmark studies in this area examined the relationship between sprawl, health behaviors, and health conditions, and involved 206,992 adults in 448 counties. It showed that people who lived in counties with greater sprawl walked less, and had higher rates of obesity and hypertension. In fact, people who lived in low sprawl areas like Manhattan and Washington, DC weighed an average of 6 pounds less than people living in high sprawl counties based on sprawl related factors.[63]

Many buildings are designed to maximize efficiency in moving from one section to another, with elevators in clear view and staircases often hidden and sometimes not very pleasant.

Large grocery stores are the predominant source of food for most people. They provide the advantage of a wide variety of food in one place, but access is sometimes limited for people who do not have cars, or who live in poor neighborhoods.

Community design and food access is governed largely by federal, state and local government laws related to transportation, zoning, agriculture, and building codes-areas that are beyond the expertise of the typical health promotion program manager, and even the leadership of many organizations. However, most employers do have control over the design of their own offices and the food served in their own cafeterias. Employers also have the choice to become more involved in shaping their environments through advocacy at the local, state and federal level.

Employers need to be aware of the impact of the built and natural environment on the health habits of their employees and either harness them or be prepared to overcome them.

E: Equality

There is a growing body of evidence that poverty has a strong impact on a wide range of health problems and that income inequality has an additional independent effect. This evidence comes to light at the same time income inequality is worse in the United States than almost any other developed nation. Additional details on the health impact of income inequality and recent increase in income disparities in the United States are shown in the Appendix B titled "Causes of Income Inequality in the United States and Resulting Health Effects."

Income inequality is relevant to workplace health promotion programs in several ways. Employees who have very low incomes or who live in states or local areas, or perhaps who work in organizations in which income inequality is high, may have elevated levels of health problems and lower levels of social trust. Additional financial resources and staff time may be required to establish trust with these employees, engage them in programs, and reverse the negative effectives of their situations. Employers need to be aware of the impact of poverty and inequality on their employees and be prepared to reduce it or overcome its effects.

Relative Importance of Different Strategies

No empirical studies have been conducted to directly test the relative importance of awareness, motivation, skills and opportunity in stimulating sustained behavior change. However, drawing from the findings of the systematic process used to develop the framework described here, I feel confident concluding that awareness is by far the least important factor, opportunities are the most important, and motivation is slightly more important than skills. One way to think about the relative importance of these factors is in the context of multivariate analysis. If these four factors could explain all the variation in successful lifestyle change, my hypothesis is that awareness would be responsible for 5% of the change, motivation for 30%, skills for 25% and opportunity for 40%. Another way to think of this is in the context of an investment portfolio; 5% of efforts and resources should be invested in enhancing awareness, 30% in enhancing motivation, 25% in building skills and 40% in providing opportunities to practice healthy lifestyles.

Conclusion and Implications

The underlying purpose of this integrated model is to create positive movement and sustained momentum for people and organizations. The five dimensions of optimal health will

The face of Wellness
A Conceptual Framework to Guide the Development of Effective Health Promotion Programs:
The Awareness, Motivation, Skills and Opportunity (AMSO) Framework and The Face of Wellness Model

capture people's attention. At worst, they will laugh and say "That's flaky." More likely, they will see the dimensions as reflecting priorities in their own life, and will look closer into programs built around these concepts. The six steps in the Renewing Health Behavior Change Process are specifically designed to keep people moving forward to building one positive behavior after another into their lives. The AMSO Portfolio Balancing Framework is designed to stimulate organizations to continually reflect on their programs to make sure they are investing the appropriate resources in areas that are most likely to make a difference, especially to stimulate people who are not health nuts...a description that probably fits most of the people reading this workbook.

Appendix A

Historical Roots of an Aspirational Vision of Health

The historical roots of an aspirational vision of health came from the early work of Bill Hettler, John Travis and Don Ardell, who came together to create the National Wellness Institute at the University of Wisconsin, Stevens Point in 1977. Hettler was a physician who directed the student health service. In 1976, he described six dimensions of wellness (Figure A-1) in a brochure intended for his student patients. These included physical, spiritual, emotional, social, intellectual and occupational health. He discussed this six-dimensional model widely in presentations, but apparently did not publish any written work on the dimensions until years after others had begun to write about it.[64] A few years earlier, apparently in 1972, John Travis, a physician and the founder of what has been described as the first wellness center in the United States, articulated a continuum of health in which premature death was shown on the left and high-level wellness on the right (Figure A-2). Traditional medicine typically focused on moving people to the mid point, helping them overcome disabilities, symptoms and signs of disease, to a point of no discernable illness, but also no discernable wellness. The emerging field of wellness would help them move through that neutral point toward high-level wellness through awareness, education and growth.[65] Early work in the health promotion field was inspired by Hetler's six dimensions of wellness and Travis's illness-wellness continuum.

The face of Wellness
A Conceptual Framework to Guide the Development of Effective Health Promotion Programs:
The Awareness, Motivation, Skills and Opportunity (AMSO) Framework and The Face of Wellness Model

Figure A-1

The Six Dimensions of Wellness

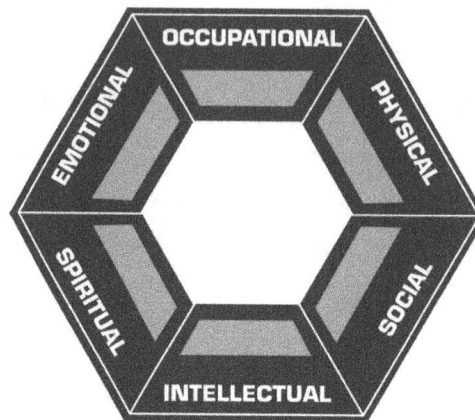

Figure A-2

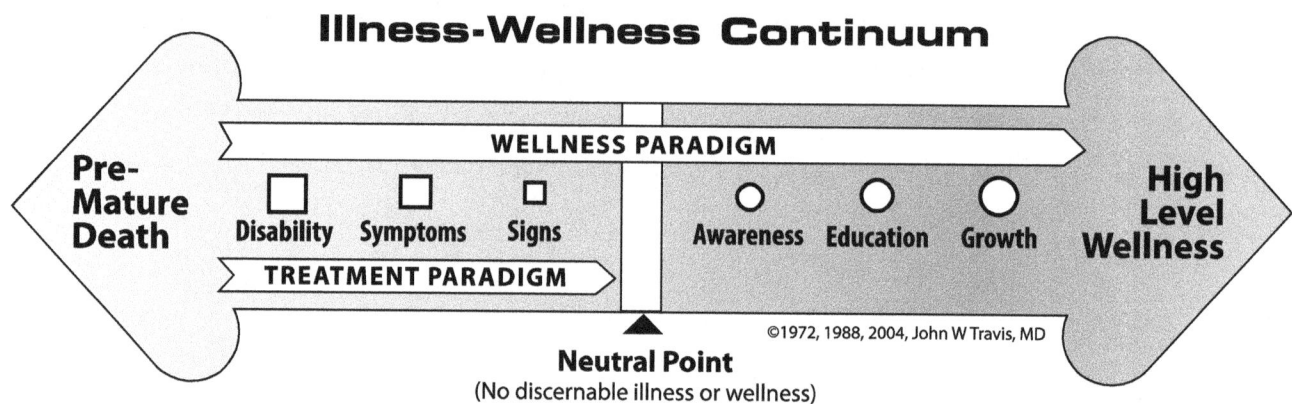

Illness-Wellness Continuum

©1972, 1988, 2004, John W Travis, MD

Neutral Point
(No discernable illness or wellness)

In 1995, O'Donnell, inspired by a personal comment from Noreen Clark, the then chairman of the Department of Health Behavior and Health Education, suggested that illness and wellness were actually not part of the same continuum and that a person did not need to pass though a point of no discernable disease to begin to move toward high-level wellness, or as he called it, optimal health.[66] For example, a person could have a terminal disease, but also be highly evolved in their emotional, spiritual, intellectual and social health. He suggested that a health matrix, with illness on one axis and wellness on the other axis, might be a more accurate conceptualization than one continuum (Figure A-3). Optimal health is shown in the top right corner of this matrix. People would strive to achieve the highest level of freedom from illness and highest level of wellness to move as close as possible to optimal health. Using this matrix better allows clinicians to better apply health promotion principles in working with sick patients. For example, despite living with the physical deterioration caused by cancer, diabetes or heart disease, there is no reason a person cannot excel in the other dimensions of optimal health. In fact, enhancing their social, intellectual, emotional and spiritual health may help them manage their physical disability. Physical activity, nutritious diet, not using tobacco or other toxic substances will facilitate recovery as well. These principles also apply to helping someone recover from an injury, heart attack or other acute but resolvable disease.

Figure A-3

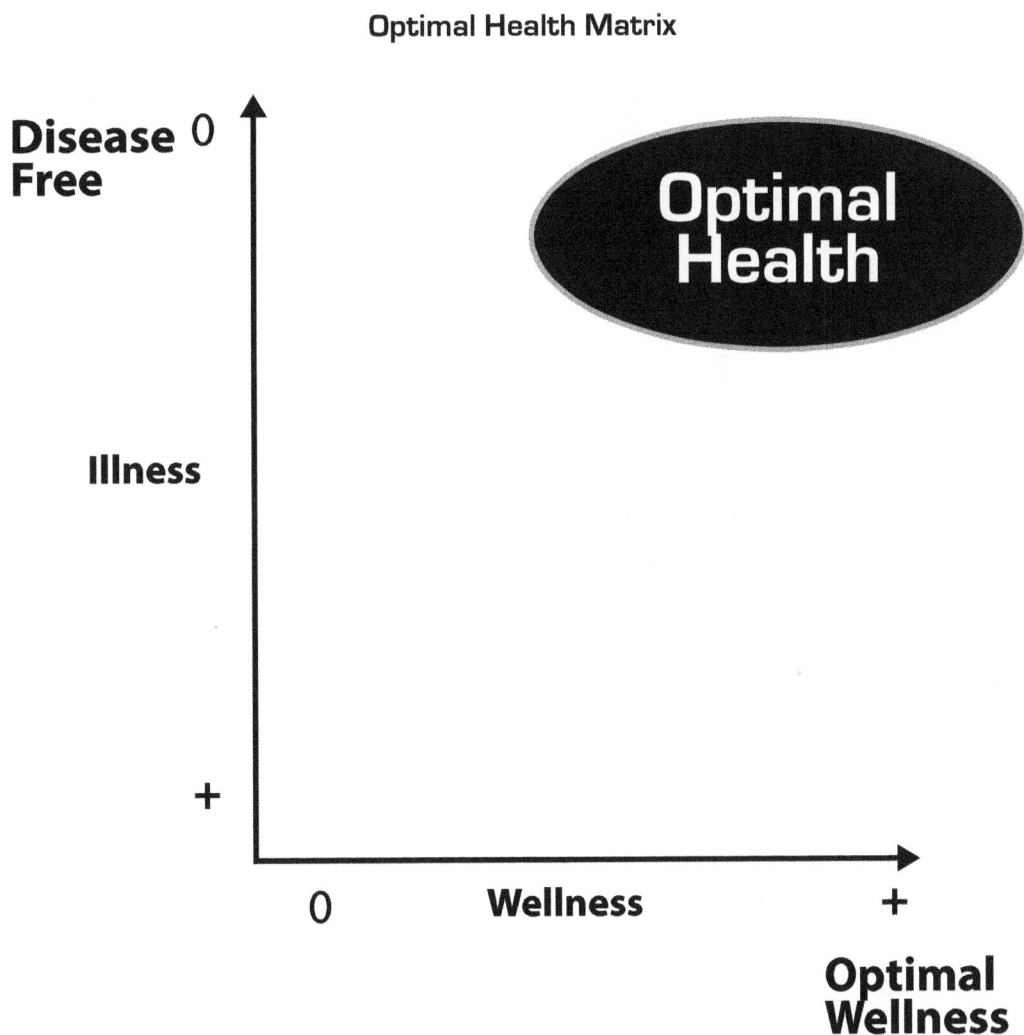

Appendix B

Causes of Income Inequality in the United States and Resulting Health Effects

Excerpt from O'Donnell MP. Erosion of Our Moral Compass, Social Trust, and the Fiscal Strength of the United States: Income Inequality, Tax Policy, and Well-Being. *Am Jour Health Promot.* 2012, 26, 4, iv-xi.

Increases in Income Disparities in the United States

The Occupy Wall Street movement [67] has focused attention on the dramatic and growing income disparities between the rich and the poor, and to a large extent between the rich and everyone else, and that the outcome of our federal spending and tax policies is to make the rich richer and the poor poorer. In fact, of the 34 nations that make up the Organization for Economic Co-operation and Development (OECD) only China, Mexico and Turkey have higher income disparities than the United States. The top 10% of Americans earn an average of $114,000/year, 15 times the $7,800 earned by the lowest 10%. The difference has gotten worse over the past 30 years; it was 12 times more in the 1990s and 10 times more in the 1980s. This disparity exists despite a 30% increase in hours worked by the lowest 10% in the past decade, and a 1% drop in hours worked by the top 1%. The income gap is more extreme for the top 1%, who earn an average of $1.3 million and collectively earn 18% of all income for the entire nation, more than two times the 8% of all income they collectively earned in 1980. During the same period, the highest marginal income tax rates in the US dropped from 70% to 35% and capital gains rates dropped from 25% to 14%; the result being that high income earners are able to keep a higher portion of the income they are earning.[68] The story on accumulated wealth is even more extreme. A recent analysis of the most current data (2007) from the Survey of Consumer Finances[69] found that the top 20% of wealth holders owns 87.2% of all the wealth in the United States, the top 1% owns 69%, and the richest 400 individuals have as much wealth as the entire bottom 50%. One family, the six heirs to the Walmart fortune, have as much wealth as the entire bottom 30% of the

The face of Wellness
A Conceptual Framework to Guide the Development of Effective Health Promotion Programs:
The Awareness, Motivation, Skills and Opportunity (AMSO) Framework and The Face of Wellness Model

population of our nation.[70] We expect to see that disparities are even more extreme when data from 2011 is released. For example, the fortune of the Walmart heirs increased from $70 billion to $93 billion between 2007 and 2011.

To exasperate the problem, the US does relatively little to help people with low income. For example, the direct financial support provided to people with low-incomes represented just 6% of their household incomes, compared to an average of 16% in the OECD nations. Spending on public services like health care and education was 13.4% of GDP, about average for the OECD nations.[71] It is shocking but not surprising that an estimated 14.7% of children in the US live in poverty, [72] despite the widely accepted finding that successful early childhood development is the best predictor of future success in life. We have also allowed the evisceration of our once great K-12 education system, seen cuts in state funding of a state college and university system that was once the envy of the world, allowed the core of many of our great cities to decay, and done little to stop the erosion of our infrastructure of roads, bridges and energy supports. Neglect in these areas hurts all of society, but has the greatest impact on those with lowest incomes.

Growing evidence of the impact of inequality on health and other aspects of quality of life.

The final factor that has made me realize I have had my head in the sand is my growing understanding of the impact of income inequality on health and other aspects of quality of life. I have learned the most in this area by reading the work of Richard Wilkinson. Richard Wilkinson is a long-time collaborator with Michael Marmot on the study of social determinants of health, and the leader of a series of studies that show the devastating impact of income inequality. The findings of these studies are described brilliantly in his book titled *The Spirit Level: Why Greater Equality Makes Societies Stronger*[73], which he co-authored with Kate Pickett. Together, they have created the Equality Trust to make these findings more visible and to rally people to look for strategies to reduce inequality. The findings from their research, slide decks and access to their original data sets are available on their website: http://www.equalitytrust.org.uk. The overall conclusion of their work is that differences in income between rich and poor, rather than per capita income per se, is one of the most powerful predictors of life expectancy, infant mortality, obesity, mental illness, teenage birth rate, homicides, imprisonment, education scores, social mobility and trust. Collectively, these factors make up an "Index of health and social problems." Their analysis begins with examining the relationship between the per capita income of a nation and life expectancy. They found that there is a strong relationship between income and life expectancy for low-income nations, with the poorest nations having life expectancies in the 40s and richer nations having life expectancies over 70. However, once per capita incomes reach about $10,000 per year, higher per capita incomes do not seem to have much impact on life expectancy. Once a per capita income has reached this baseline level, income inequality is more important than per capita income in explaining life expectancy. Most of their global analysis is based on 23 nations. They started with the 50 wealthiest nations of the world, dropped those with populations of less than 3 million people and those that did not have good data on income inequity and the other outcome variables in their analysis, which is described below.

They have analyzed and reported these relationships for their sample of 23 nations and for the 50 states in the United States. The strength of the relationships is remarkably strong, reaching statistical significance for all of these outcomes, and explaining 18% to 86% of the variances in the individual factors and 76% of the variance in the Index of health and social problems. Using data from the developed nations, but not from the individual US states, they found statistically significant relationships between income inequality and drug use, calorie intake, child well-being, juvenile homicides, child mental illness, public expenditures on health care, paid maternity leave, child conflict, recycling, peace index, spending on police, social expenditures, women's status, high school dropout, pugnacity and spending on foreign aid.

The consistency of these relationships is remarkable. Variances of this magnitude mean that income inequality is an important predictor for all these outcomes, and probably the most important factor for some of them. I was stunned, and quite frankly ashamed, that the United States ranked so poorly on so many of these values. This certainly does not jive with the view so many Americans hold, including me, that the United States is the greatest nation in the world. It leaves me trying to think of the ways in which we are the greatest, and quit frankly, after reading this work, I am challenged in that task. The biggest shock for me was how poorly we rank in foreign aid as a percent of GDP...dead last among the 23 nations in their study! We are also the worst in income inequality, social mobility, and the rates of imprisonment, teenage births, mental illness, obesity, homicides, infant mortality, and overweight children. In addition, the US is almost the worst in illegal drug use, child well-being, educational testing scores, child conflict, recycling, ecological footprint and life expectancy.

The face of Wellness
A Conceptual Framework to Guide the Development of Effective Health Promotion Programs:
The Awareness, Motivation, Skills and Opportunity (AMSO) Framework and The Face of Wellness Model

We are about average on women's status and the level of trust. The only areas the US ranks at the top are income per capita, military spending per capita and medical care spending per capita.

Damaging effects of inequality

Why does inequality have such a strong impact? Inequality seems to have a devastating and cascading effect on health and other factors for at least five reasons.

First, poverty, independent of inequality, causes many health problems. These problems leave poor people with lower resilience to recover from the additional risks caused by inequality. For example, medical conditions that are higher for people with low income include obesity,[74] asthma,[75] diabetes,[76] hypertension,[77] human immunodeficiency virus infection,[78] and coronary heart disease and stroke,[79] as well as preterm birth [80] and adolescent pregnancy.[81] Smoking rates are higher among people with lower incomes and less education,[82] as are death by homicide[83] and premature death by any cause. Rates of disease and death are higher for these groups partly because of poor health habits, but also because of lack of access to clean and safe housing[84] and clean air, [85] and poor access to regular medical care,[86] nutritious foods, and formal education.[87]

Second, inequality causes people to judge themselves negatively relative to other people, a phenomenon called "social evaluative threat" which in turn has been shown to trigger release of cortisol and proinflammatory cytokine.[88] Cortisol impedes immune functions, increases the risk of heart disease and threatens other physiological systems. Chronic inflammation has been linked to increased rates of autoimmune disorders including rheumatoid arthritis, lupus and polymyalgia rheumatica, asthma and the inflammatory bowel diseases ulcerative colitis, Crohn's disease, cardiovascular disease, bacterial endocarditis, cancer, urinary infections or cystitis and may increase risk of a squamous cell bladder cancer.[89] An indirect impact of social evaluative threat is that defending one's honor becomes more important, and can lead to physical injuries caused by fighting and the additional stress caused by hostile interactions.

Third, the importance of maintaining status increases the social pressure to divert limited financial resources from food, rent, utilities, medical care and other necessities of basic living that will preserve good health, to buying nice clothes, cars, toys for kids or entertainment to raise status, or to drugs, alcohol or cigarettes to help cope with the stress. This temptation to divert resources from basic needs to entertainment and luxuries is much lower in poor nations in which incomes are low for all people because these discretionary luxuries are rare, not promoted through ubiquitous advertising and rarely purchased by peers. As such, the standard of living a typical family in a poor nation that has low levels of income inequality might be similar to the standard of living of a poor person in the United States (which has high income inequality) in an absolute sense, but the person living in the poor nation does not suffer the negative consequences of income inequality because their standard of living is the same as everyone else they encounter.

Fourth, a pregnant woman experiencing the elevated stress caused by inequality generates cortisol and other stress related hormones and toxins. This combination can cause lasting damage to her fetus, increasing the likelihood of low birth weight, premature birth, or other congenital defects. This is in addition to the damage to the fetus caused by malnutrition. This makes it very difficult for this woman's child to ever catch up.

Fifth, early childhood development is impacted directly by poverty. For example, Goodman and Gregg found that the most important factors affecting child development are birth weight, mother suffering from post-natal depression, being read to every day at age 3 and having a regular bed time at age three,[90] and that all of those factors are related to socio-economic status. Recovering from these setbacks compounds the challenges of a child born into poverty. For example, one of the findings of the 1970 British Cohort Study was that children in high socioeconomic (SES) status families maintained or improved their cognitive abilities relative to their peers as time passed, while those from low SES families dropped. More specifically, a cohort of children from high SES family who tested at the 10th percentile at 22 months, averaged scores at the 55th percentile at 118 months, while those from low SES families averaged scores at the 28th percentile at 118 months. Similarly, high SES children who tested at 90th percentile at 22 months, averaged scores at the 68th percentile at 118 months while low SES children averaged scores at the 39th percentile at 118 months.[91] It is important to acknowledge the racial bias in cognitive testing in interpreting these findings, [92] but it is hard to not conclude that poverty has a depressing impact on cognitive development. This childhood development effect is exasperated by the fact that social standing and peer acceptance is especially important to adolescent children. Those with depressed

The face of Wellness
A Conceptual Framework to Guide the Development of Effective Health Promotion Programs:
The Awareness, Motivation, Skills and Opportunity (AMSO) Framework and The Face of Wellness Model

cognitive development tend to have lower social status, which produces more stress and the physical problems caused by stress, as well as increased temptation to perform risky behaviors to get attention or join gangs to enhance social relationships.

Racial discrimination is no doubt closely aligned with income inequality. Wilkinson does not specifically address racial discrimination in his book and a thorough review of this is beyond the scope of this paper, but a few key points need to be acknowledged. The most obvious link between income inequality and racial discrimination is that oppressed racial groups have lower incomes, [93] and thus suffer from all the negative income inequality effects described above. In addition, some people are victims of discrimination because of their race, independent of their income. In addition to increased threats of violence and exclusion from many opportunities, this discrimination creates the same type of stress caused by social evaluative threat, and the resulting physical consequences. For people with high and middle incomes who suffer racial discrimination, this subjects them to stresses they would otherwise be able to avoid. For people with low income, it increases the stress they already endure from poverty and income inequality.

References

1   O'Donnell MP, Bishop CA, Kaplan KL. Benchmarking best practices in workplace health promotion. *Am J Health Promot.* 1996:11[4]:TAHP-1–TAHP-8.

2   O'Donnell MP. Health impact of workplace health promotion programs and methodological quality of the research literature. *Art Health Promot.* 1997;1:1–7.

3   Wilson MG, Holman PB, Hammock A. A comprehensive review of the effects of worksite health promotion on health-related outcomes. *Am J Health Promot.* 1996;10:429–435.

4   Wilson MG. A comprehensive review of the effects of worksite health promotion on health-related outcomes: an update. *Am J Health Promot.* 1996;11:107–108.

5   Aldana SG. Financial impact of health promotion programs: a comprehensive review of the literature. *Am J Health Promot.* 2001;15:296-320.

6   The Health Project Web site. C. Everett Koop Award Winners. Available at: http://www.thehealthproject.com/index.html. Accessed August 15, 2012.

7   O'Donnell MP. Definition of health promotion. *Am J Health Promot.* 1986;1:3.

8   Naditch MP. The StayWell Program. In: *Behavioral Health.* New York: John Wiley & Sons; 1984:1071–1078.

9   The Twelve Traditions. *AA Grapevine.* 1949:6[6].

10   Prochaska JO, Velicer WF. The transtheoretical model of health behavior change. *Am J Health Promot.* 1997;12:38-48.

11   National Heart Lung and Blood Institute. Diseases and conditions index Web site. Available at: http://www.nhlbi.nih.gov/health/dci/Diseases/ms/ms_whatis.html. Accessed October 1, 2012.

12   Heaney C, Goetzel R. A review of health-related outcomes of multi-component worksite health promotion programs. *Am J Health Promot.* 1997;11:290-307.

13   Rothkopf E, Billington M. Goal-guided learning from text: inferring a descriptive processing model from inspection times and eye movements. *J Educ Psychol.* 1979;71:310–327.

14   Bryan J, Locke E. Goal setting as a means of increasing motivation. *J Appl Psychol.* 1967;51:274–277.

15   LaPorte R, Nath R. Role of performance goals in prose learning. *J Educ Psychol.* 1976;68:260–264.

The face of Wellness
A Conceptual Framework to Guide the Development of Effective Health Promotion Programs:
The Awareness, Motivation, Skills and Opportunity (AMSO) Framework and The Face of Wellness Model

16   Wood R, Locke E. Goal setting and strategy effects on complex tasks. In: Staw B, Cummings L, eds. *Research in Organizational Behavior.* Vol 12. Greenwich, Conn: JAI Press; 1990:73–109.

17   Seijts GH, Latham GP, Tasa K, Latham BW. Goal setting and goal orientation: an integration of two different yet related literatures. *Acad Manage J.* 2004;47:227–239.

18   Kanfer R, Aclerman PL. Motivation and cognitive abilities: an integrative/aptitude-treatment interaction approach to skill acquisition. *J Appl Psychol.* 1989;74:657-690.

19   Seijts GH, Latham GP. The effect of distal learning, outcome, and proximal goals on a moderately complex task. *J Organ Behav.* 2001;22:291–302.

20   Locke EA, Latham GP. A theory of goal setting and task performance. Englewood Cliffs, NJ: Prentice Hall; 1990.

21   Wagner J, Gooding R. Effects of societal trends on participation research. *Adm Sci Q.* 1987;32:241–262.

22   Locke EA, Alavi M, Wagner J. Participation in decision-making: an information exchange perspective. In: Ferris G, ed. *Research in Personnel and Human Resources Management.* Vol 15. Greenwich, CT: JAI Press; 1997:293–331.

23   Hollenbeck J, Williams C, Klein H. An empirical examination of the antecedents of commitment to difficult goals. *J Appl Psychol.* 1989;74:18–23.

24   Roman WW, Latham GP, Kinne SB. The effects of goal setting and supervision on worker behavior in an industrial situation. *J Appl Psychol.* 1973;58:302–207.

25   Bandura A. *Self-Efficacy: The Exercise of Control.* New York, NY: Freeman; 1997.

26   Matsui T, Okada A, Inoshita O. Mechanism of feedback affecting task performance. *Organ Behav Hum Perform.* 1983;31:114–122.

27   US Dept of Health and Human Services, Office of the Surgeon General. Clinical practice guideline: treating tobacco use and dependence: 2008 update. Available at: http://www.surgeon-general.gov/tobacco/treating_tobacco_use08.pdf. Accessed August 30, 2012.

28   Bandura A. Self-efficacy: toward a unifying theory of behavior change. *Psychol Rev.* 1977;84:191–215.

29   Brown LB, Neese RM, Vinokur AD, Smith DM. Providing social support may be more beneficial than receiving it: results from a prospective study of mortality. *Psychol Sci.* 2003;14:320–327.

30   O'Donnell MP, Ainsworth T. *Health Promotion in the Workplace.* Albany, New York: John Wiley and Sons; 1984.

31   O'Donnell MP. A simple framework to describe what works best: improving awareness, enhancing motivation, building skills, and providing opportunity. *Am J Health Promot.* 2005;20: suppl 1-7 following 84, iii.

32   Aizen I. From intentions to actions: a theory of planned behavior in action. In: Kiehl J, Bechman J, eds. *Action Control: From Cognition to Behavior.* New York, NY: Springer-Verlag; 1985:11–39.

33   Prochaska J, Velicer W. The transtheoretical model of health behavior change. *Am J Health Promot.* 1997;12:38–48.

34   Koffman D, Lee J, Hopp J, Emont S. The impact of including incentives and competition in a workplace smoking cessation program on quit rates. *Am J Health Promot.* 1998;13:105–111.

35   Taitel MS, Haufle V, Heck D, et al. Incentives and other factors associated with employee participation in health risk assessment. *J Occup Environ Med.* 2008;50:863–872.

36   Seaverson EL, Grossmeier J, Miller TM, Anderson DR. The role of incentive design, incentive, value, communications strategy, and worksite culture on health risk assessment participation. *Am J Health Promot.* 2009;23:343-352.

37   Towers Watson. 2011/2012 Staying@Work survey report: a pathway to employee health and workplace productivity. Available at: http://www.towerswatson.com/united-states/research/6031. Accessed August 16, 2012.

38   Miller W, Rolnick S. *Motivational Interviewing: Preparing People to Change Addictive Behavior.* New York, NY: Guilford; 1991.

39   O'Donnell MP, Harris JS. *Health Promotion in the Workplace.* 2nd ed. Albany, NY: Delmar Publishers; 1994.

40   O'Donnell MP. *Health Promotion in the Workplace.* 3rd ed. Albany, NY: Cenage; 2002.

41   Posse. Merriam-Webster dictionary Web site. Available at: http://www.merriam-webster.com/dictionary/posse. Accessed August 31, 2012

42   Posse. Urban Dictionary Web site. Available at: http://www.urbandictionary.com/define.php?term=posse. Accessed August 31, 2012.

43   Framingham Heart Study Web site. Available at: http://www.framinghamheartstudy.org/. Accessed August 31, 2012.

44   Christakis NA, Fowler JH. The spread of obesity in a large social network over 32 years. [published online ahead of print July 25, 2007]. *N Engl J Med.* 2007;357:370–379.

45   Christakis NA, Fowler JH. The collective dynamics of smoking in a large social network. *N Engl J Med.* 2008;358:2249–2258.

46   Rosenquist JN, Fowler JH, Christakis NA. Social network determinants of depression [published online ahead of print March 16, 2010]. *Mol Psychiatry.* 2011;16:273–281.

47   Rosenquist JN, Murabito J, Fowler JH, Christakis NA. The spread of alcohol consumption behavior in a large social network. *Ann Intern Med.* 2010;152:426–433, W141.

The face of Wellness
A Conceptual Framework to Guide the Development of Effective Health Promotion Programs:
The Awareness, Motivation, Skills and Opportunity (AMSO) Framework and The Face of Wellness Model

48   O'Donnell MP. Integrating health promotion in the national agenda: the pers-pective of a grass roots advocate. *Health Educ Behav.* 2012;39:518-22.

49   US state and local issues. Campaign for Tobacco Free Kids Web site. Available at: http://www.tobaccofreekids.org/what_we_do/state_local/. Accessed August 17, 2012.

50   O'Donnell MP. Fool me once, shame on you. Fool me twice, shame on me [Editor's Notes]. *Am J Health Promot.* 2008;23:iv.

51   New York City Dept of Health and Mental Hygiene Web site. Available at: http://www.nyc.gov/html/doh/html/home/home.shtml. Accessed August 17, 2012.

52   Running USA's A-nnual Marathon Report. Available at: http://www.runningusa.org/index.cfm?fuseaction=news.details&ArticleId=332&returnTo=annual-reports. Accessed August 20, 2012.

53   The health consequences of involuntary exposure to tobacco smoke: a report of the Surgeon General. Atlanta, GA: US Dept of Health and Human Services, Centers for Disease Control and Prevention, Coordinating Center for Health Promotion, National Center for Chronic Disease Prevention and Health Promotion, Office on Smoking and Health; 2006.

54   State smoke-free laws for worksites, restaurants, and bars—United States, 2000-2010. *MMWR Morb Mortal Wkly Rep.* 2011:60;472–475. Available at: http://www.cdc.gov/mmwr/preview/mmwrhtml/mm6015a2.htm#tab1. Accessed October 1, 2012.

55   American Nonsmokers Rights Foundation. Summary of 100% smokefree state laws and population protected by 100% US smokefree laws, July 1, 2012. Available at: http://www.no-smoke.org/pdf/SummaryUSPopList.pdf. Accessed October 1, 2012.

56   Giovino GA, Chaloupka FJ, Hartman AM, et al. Cigarette smoking prevalence and policies in the 50 states: an era of change—the Robert Wood Johnson Foundation ImpacTeen Tobacco Chart Book. Buffalo, NY: University at Buffalo, State University of New York; 2009. Available at: http://impacteen.org/statetobaccodata/chartbook_final060409.pdf. Accessed August 20, 2012.

57   Baezconde-Garbanati LA, Weich-Reushé K, Espinoza L, et al. Secondhand smoke exposure among Hispanics/Latinos living in multiunit housing: exploring barriers to new policies. *Am J Health Promot.* 2011;25(5 suppl):S82–S90.

58   Oprah's weight loss confession. Available at: http://www.oprah.com/health/Oprahs-Weight-Loss-Confession/. Accessed August 20, 2012.

59   National Eating Disorders Web site. Available at: http://www.nationaleating-disorders.org/. Accessed August 20, 2012.

[60]   Active Living by Design Web site. Available at: http://www.activelivingbydesign.org/. Accessed August 20, 2012.

[61]   Active Living Research. Available at: http://www.activelivingresearch.org/. Accessed August 20, 2012.

[62]   Healthy Eating Research Web site. Available at: http://www.healthyeatingresearch.org/. Accessed August 20, 2012.

[63]   Ewing R, Schmid T, Killingsworth R, et al. Relationship between urban sprawl and physical activity, obesity, and morbidity. *Am J Health Promot.* 2003;18:47–57.

[64]   National Wellness Institute. The six dimensions of wellness model. Available at: http://www.nationalwellness.org/index.php?id_tier=2&id_c=25. Accessed August 30, 2012

[65]   Ardell D. Meet John Travis, doctor of wellbeing. *Prevention.* 1975;4:62–69.

[66]   O'Donnell MP. *How to Design Workplace Health Promotion Programs.* Keego Harbor, MI: American Journal of Health Promotion, Inc; 1995.

[67]   Occupy Wall Street. The revolution continues world wide. Available at: http://occupy-wallst.org/. Accessed December 22, 2011.

[68]   Congressional Budget Office. Trends in federal tax revenues and rate, December 2, 2010. Available at: http://www.cbo.gov/doc.cfm?index=11976. Accessed October 1, 2012.

[69]   Board of Governors of the Federal Reserve. Survey of consumer finances. Available at: http://www.federalreserve.gov/econresdata/scf/scf_2009p.htm. Accessed December 12, 2011.

[70]   Allegretto S. The few, the proud, the very rich. Center on Wage and Employment Dynamics. December 5, 2011. Available at: http://blogs.berkeley.edu/2011/12/05/the-few-the-proud-the-very-rich/. Accessed December 12, 2011.

[71]   Organization for Economic Co-operation and Development. Divided we stand: why inequality keeps rising. December 2011. Available at: http://www.oecd.org/document/51/0,3746, en_2649_33933_49147827_1_1_1_1,00.html. Accessed October 1, 2012.

[72]   Annie E. Casey Foundation. Promoting opportunity for the next generation, 2011 KIDS COUNT data book. State profiles of child well-being. Available at: http://www.aecf.org//media/Pubs/Initiatives/KIDS%20COUNT/123/2011KIDSCOUNTDataBook/KCDataBook2011.pdf. Accessed August 23, 2011.

[73]   Wilkinson R, Pickett K. *The Spirit Level: Why Greater Equality Makes Societies Stronger.* New York, NY: Bloomberg Press; 2009.

[74]   Freedman DS. Obesity—United States, *1988–2008. MMWR Morb Mortal Wkly Rep.* 2011;60(suppl):73–77. Available at: http://www.cdc.gov/mmwr/pdf/other/su6001.pdf. Accessed August 23, 2011.

The face of Wellness
A Conceptual Framework to Guide the Development of Effective Health Promotion Programs:
The Awareness, Motivation, Skills and Opportunity (AMSO) Framework and The Face of Wellness Model

[75]   Moorman JE, Zahran H, Truman BI, Molla MT. Current asthma prevalence—United States, 2006-2008. *MMWR Morb Mortal Wkly Rep.* 2011;60(suppl):84-86. Available at: http://www.cdc.gov/mmwr/pdf/other/su6001.pdf. Accessed August 23, 2011.

[76]   Beckles GL, Zhu J, Moonesinghe R. Diabetes—United States, 2004 and 2008. *MMWR Morb Mortal Wkly Rep.* 2011;60(suppl):90-93. Available at: http://www.cdc.gov/mmwr/pdf/other/su6001.pdf. Accessed August 23, 2011.

[77]   Keenan NL, Rosendorf KA. Prevalence of hypertension and controlled hypertension—United States, 2005-2008. *MMWR Morb Mortal Wkly Rep.* 2011;60(suppl):94-98. Available at: http://www.cdc.gov/mmwr/pdf/other/su6001.pdf. Accessed August 23, 2011.

[78]   Hughes D, Dean HD, Mermin J. H. Fenton KA. HIV infection—United States, 2005 and 2008. *MMWR Morb Mortal Wkly Rep.* 2011;60(suppl):87-89. Available at: http://www.cdc.gov/mmwr/pdf/other/su6001.pdf. Accessed August 23, 2011.

[79]   Keenan NL, Shaw KM. Coronary heart disease and stroke deaths—United States, 2006. *MMWR Morb Mortal Wkly Rep.* 2011;60(suppl):62-66. Available at: http://www.cdc.gov/mmwr/pdf/other/su6001.pdf. Accessed August 23, 2011.

[80]   Martin JA. Preterm births—United States, 2007. *MMWR Morb Mortal Wkly Rep.* 2011;60(suppl):78-79. Available at: http://www.cdc.gov/mmwr/pdf/other/su6001.pdf. Accessed August 23, 2011.

[81]   Ventura SJ. Adolescent pregnancy and childbirth—United States, 1991-2008. *MMWR Morb Mortal Wkly Rep.* 2011;60(suppl):105-109. Available at: http://www.cdc.gov/mmwr/pdf/other/su6001.pdf. Accessed August 23, 2011.

[82]   Garrett BE. Cigarette smoking—United States, 1965-2008. *MMWR Morb Mortal Wkly Rep.* 2011;60(suppl):109-113. Available at: http://www.cdc.gov/mmwr/pdf/other/su6001.pdf. Accessed August 23, 2011.

[83]   Logan JE, Smith SG, Stevens MR. Homicides—United States, 1999-2007. *MMWR Morb Mortal Wkly Rep.* 2011;60(suppl):67-72. Available at: http://www.cdc.gov/mmwr/pdf/other/su6001.pdf. Accessed August 23, 2011.

[84]   Raymond J, Wheeler W, Brown MJ. Inadequate and unhealthy housing, 2007 and 2009. *MMWR Morb Mortal Wkly Rep.* 2011;60(suppl):21-27. Available at: http://www.cdc.gov/mmwr/pdf/other/su6001.pdf. Accessed August 23, 2011.

[85]   Yip FY, Pearcy JN, Garbe PL, Truman BI. Unhealthy air quality—United States, 2006-2009. *MMWR Morb Mortal Wkly Rep.* 2011;60(suppl):28-31. Available at: http://www.cdc.gov/mmwr/pdf/other/su6001.pdf. Accessed August 23, 2011.

[86]   Moonesinghe R, Zhu J, Truman BI. Health insurance coverage—United States, 2004 and 2008. *MMWR Morb Mortal Wkly Rep.* 2011;60(suppl):35-37. Available at: http://www.cdc.gov/mmwr/pdf/other/su6001.pdf. Accessed August 23, 2011.

[87]   Beckles GL, Truman BI. Education and income—United States, 2005 and 2009. *MMWR Morb Mortal Wkly Rep.* 2011;60(suppl):13-17. Available at: http://www.cdc.gov/mmwr/pdf/other/su6001.pdf. Accessed August 23, 2011.

[88]   Dickerson SS. Emotional and physiological responses to social-evaluative threat. *Soc Pers Psychol Compass* [serial online]. Blackwell. March 2008. Available at: http://www.blackwell-compass.com/subject/socialpsychology/article_view?article_id=spco_articles_bpl095. Accessed January 6, 2012.

[89]   Leserman J, Petitto JM, Golden RN, Gaynes BN, et al. Impact of stressful life events, depression, social support, coping, and cortisol on progression to AIDS. *Am J Psychiatry.* 2000;157:1221-1228. doi:10.1176/appi.ajp.157.8.1221. Available at: http://ajp.psychiatryonline.org/article.aspx?articleID=174261. Accessed January 6, 2012.

[90]   Goodman A, Gregg P, Washburn E. Children's educational attainment and the aspirations, attitudes and behaviours of parents and children through childhood in the UK. *Longit Life Course Stud.* 2011;2:1-18.

[91]   Feinstein L. Inequality in the early cognitive development of British children in the 1970 cohort. *Economica.* 2003;70:3-97.

[92]   Morgan ATA, Marsiske M, Dzierzewski J, et al. Race-related cognitive test bias in the ACTIVE study: a MIMIC model approach. *Exp Aging Res.* 2010;36:426-452. Available at: http://www.ncbi.nlm.nih.gov/pmc/articles/PMC2941916/. Accessed January 6, 2010.

[93]   US Census Bureau. Income, expenditures, poverty, & wealth, the 2012 statistical abstract. Available at: http://www.census.gov/compendia/statab/cats/income_expenditures_poverty_wealth.html. Accessed January 6, 2012.

About the Author

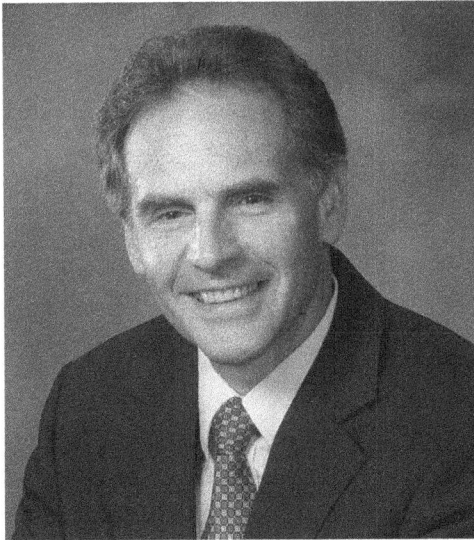

Dr. O'Donnell is the Director of the Health Management Research Center in the School of Kinesiology of the University of Michigan. Formed in 1978, the Center has helped more than 1000 work-sites measure the health risks of their employees; calculate the link between health risks, medical costs and productivity; evaluate the impact of their health promotion programs; and in the process, establish the scientific foundation for this area of research. Dr. O'Donnell has worked directly with employers, health care organizations, government agencies, founda-tions, insurance companies and health promotion providers to develop new and refine existing health promotion programs and has served in leadership roles in four major health systems. He is Founder, President and Editor-in-Chief of the *American Journal of Health Promotion* and is also Founder and Chairman Emeritus of Health Promotion Advocates, a non-profit policy group created to integrate health promo-tion strategies into national policy. Health Promotion Advocates was successful in develop-ing six provisions that became law as part of the Affordable Care Act. He has co-authored 6 books and workbooks, including *Health Promotion in the Workplace,* which was in continuous publication for 27 years, and more than 190 articles, book chapters and columns. He has presented more than 260 keynote and workshop presentations on six continents, served on boards and committees for 48 non-profit and for-profit organizations and received 13 national awards. His most recent awards are the Elizabeth Fries Health Education Award presented by the James F. and Sarah T. Fries Foundation, and the Bill Whitmer Leadership Award, presented by the Health Enhancement Research Organization (HERO). He earned a PhD in Health Behavior from University of Michigan, an MBA in General Management and an MPH in Hospital Management, both from University of California, Berkeley, and an AB in psychobiology from Oberlin College. He attended high school and was later a Senior Fulbright Scholar and visiting professor in Seoul, South Korea.